Understanding Metabolism

The Truth About Counting Calories, Sustainable Weight Loss, and Metabolic Damage

by Scott Abel

Published by:

Scott Abel

Copyright © 2015 – Scott Abel

ISBN-13: 978-1514759165
ISBN-10: 1514759160

ALL RIGHTS RESERVED. No part of this publication may be reproduced or transmitted in any form whatsoever, electronic, or mechanical, including photocopying, recording, or by any informational storage or retrieval system without express written, dated and signed permission from the author.

Table of Contents

About the Author 7

Introduction 9

PART 1
What You Need To Know To Lose Weight
...And KEEP It Off!

Chapter 1.
A Calorie Is Not A Calorie 19

Chapter 2.
Calorie Math 27

Chapter 3.
The Metabolic Compensation System 33

Chapter 4.
Metabolic Damage 41

Chapter 5.
More Research on Metabolic Damage 49

Chapter 6.
Restoring and Repairing a Damaged
Metabolism 59

Chapter 7.
Exercise I: Quality Over Quantity 71

Chapter 8.
Exercise II: How Cardio Can Make You Fat 79

Chapter 9.
Dieting As You Get Older 87

Chapter 10.
Stress and Metabolism 93

Chapter 11.
Seven Magic Words For a Healthy Metabolism 99

Chapter 12.
Routine and Structure 111

PART 2
Diet Trends And Diet Truths

Chapter 13.
Metabolic Typing 121

Chapter 14.
Realistic Protein Needs 125

Chapter 15.
On Paleo I 131

Chapter 16.
Paleo II 138

Chapter 17.
The REAL "Low-Carb" Diet 145

Chapter 18.
Gluten...157

Chapter 19.
The Lowly Potato 163

Chapter 20.
The Truth About Coffee 173

Chapter 21.
Artificial Sweeteners 181

Chapter 22.
How to Spot Diet Scams 189

Learn More 197

About the Author

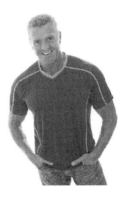

Scott Abel has been involved in the diet, fitness, and bodybuilding industries for over four decades. He has written for, or been featured in magazines like Muscle & Fitness, Flex, Muscle Mag, T-Nation, and many more.

Understanding Metabolism is about the factors that affect human metabolism, the truth about calories, nutrition, and metabolic damage, and what you need to know to lose weight and keep it off.

Introduction

by M. R. Forest

Scott asked me to write an introduction to his new book, *Understanding Metabolism*, since I've been working closely with him to get it together and ready for publication. I've been a client of Scott's, I've purchased many of his products, and I actually now work with him on his website and his publishing.

Suffice it to say, I like Scott's work and his approach a whole lot. Namely, he mixes academic research and his decades of experience, and balances that out by never losing sight of the real-world context of a situation.

It's in this way that this book in particular is a continuation or even a kind of "prequel" to Scott's previously published book, *Beyond Metabolism*.

One of the themes in *Beyond Metabolism* is the idea that your food or eating issues are, despite what you might think, not always strictly "metabolic" in nature, so we need to stop thinking strictly in those terms. Often everything related to health and weight loss is compartmentalized into how well your "training" and your "diet" are going, but obviously real life, health and fitness don't really work that way. Our current issues with weight gain, and weight *re*-gain, also have to do with the way our brains are wired, and the way our hunger and satiety feedback loops didn't evolve to deal with our modern culture of abundance, the hyper-palatable foods that are sold to us, and the environmental cues that surround us, all of which tell us to "feel" hungry, even if we are not. More than anything, the book argues, what we need to do is expand our scope, and consider a wider context when looking at such issues: we need to go "beyond" metabolism.

Although this new book is a sort of prequel, and although this new book really *is* about "metabolism," *Understanding Metabolism* continues many of those same themes, arguing that we need less "micro" analysis, more "macro" analysis, and more consideration of context. Put simply, your metabolism doesn't exist in isolation. It interacts with other elements of your biology, and even your modern environment.

Even when focusing solely on metabolism as such, we need to expand our view of the bigger picture, not focus on tinier and tinier details like nutrient timing, post-workout shakes, what time to stop eating at night, or whatever the current vogue trend is.

Sure, the laws of thermodynamics are true, and you will never gain weight if you "eat 1,500 calories but burn

2,000." Of course that is true, technically speaking. No one who says "a calorie is not a calorie" actually believes there is some secret magic voodoo that somehow overrides the laws of basic physics. They simply believe that when we think of metabolism in a real-world context, we need to go beyond a daily estimate of some static calories in/calories out equation, and appreciate the dynamic nature of the various processes that make up human metabolism.

Since metabolism is dynamic, you won't ever burn exactly 2,000 calories, day in and day out, forever and ever. Moreover, the 1,500 calories you *do* eat will affect both how much you burn, and how those calories you burn are used. (Tissue building? Fat storage? What will they do for mood or energy levels? How will they affect satiety?) Scott argues that to think that "metabolism" can be reduced to the number of calories you burn or store each day is a mistake, because of the sheer complexity and dynamism of your metabolism, and all the factors that affect it.

Understanding Metabolism is not a textbook (though references are often included, for the curious), and you don't need an advanced degree in nutrition to understand anything you read here.

In fact, chapter 11 of part one of this book uses just one simple phrase — seven words — to sum up how to keep a metabolism healthy. Keeping a metabolism working as it should doesn't need to be complicated, or require fancy formulas or specific timing of nutrients or whatever.

Scott's main aim in this book is to give you both general information and practical advice to help you keep your metabolism healthy, or identify a damaged metabolism. If yours *is* already damaged, there is information and guidance to begin its healing process. Sometimes that means tough love, but as Scott emphasizes to his coaching clients: a good coach must always, *always* be in your corner, and have your health first and foremost in their mind. No exceptions. Remember that, and you'll see where he's coming from.

You'll find a secondary aim here too: to dismantle certain ideas in the fitness industry that Scott finds extremely damaging, especially for people's metabolisms and longterm metabolic health.

In his practice as a fitness and physique coach, many of Scott's clients come to him with metabolisms damaged by ill-conceived ideas about what they've been told is "healthy," or ideas about the best way to lose weight. Or, sometimes they've just had a poor coach in the past who's put them on insane diets and ridiculous cardio regimens for the sake of short-term success (so the coach can boast about some ridiculous 12-week transformation), all at the expense of actual longterm metabolic health. It's short-sighted. Reading this book, you'll get the sense, as I did, that Scott is downright tired of some of the damaging advice that's being given out there.

You absolutely can work with your metabolism to lose weight. What you *cannot* do, and what Scott consistently warns you about, is work "against" it. A short-term diet, a "12-week miracle diet," or a cleanse or "quick start" diet, is not *really* going to help you, metabolically speaking, nor help you with actual, sustainable weight loss. You want to train your metabolism to be cooperative, not experience a "bit" of short-term weight loss at the expense of longterm metabolic and hormonal health.

One of the key ideas you'll find throughout this book is the idea that you have to learn to work *with* your body, and you do have to think long-term.

When it comes to weight loss, progress is never 100% linear, and anyone who promises you that is trying to sell you something. (This is one of Scott's principles of how to spot a diet scam, in the book's final chapter.) This is doubly the case with your metabolism, where sometimes you need to sacrifice short-term cosmetic goals (like losing 10 lbs *right this instant*) for longterm metabolic health and long-term *sustainable* weight loss. Yes, you can lose those 10 lbs right now with some insane, deprivation diet, but if you do, you'll just gain that weight back, and your metabolism will be the worse for it, and things'll be even harder for you next time. If you want to lose weight and actually *keep it off*, you need to have a cooperative metabolism, not one that is forced to compensate against what it can only perceive as starvation.

This means that often the shortest path to your ultimate goal is counter-intuitive. If your metabolism is compromised, you need to lay off overdoing the exercise, especially the cardio, and stop counting calories or trying to diet your way through what the research calls metabolic dysregulation (or, in layman's terms: "metabolic hell").

In the first few chapters Scott discusses why a calorie is not a calorie, and why calorie math doesn't add up. Calorie math might seem to work for a short-term "12-week transformation" or something, but if you want a healthy and cooperative metabolism, and you want the weight to stay off, the picture looks different. Scott calls this the "biology of weight control," and it is not what is being sold to you.

From there Scott moves on to discussing your body's metabolic compensation system, and why metabolic damage occurs, what it looks like, and what you should and should *not* do about it. The tricky thing here is not so much that there are a lot of myths in the industry about this, but that the solutions can be counter-intuitive, and they might not be what will make you "feel" productive or even like you are making progress.

Scott then discusses what "healthy" eating looks like, in terms of metabolic health, and some strategies for keeping a metabolism healthy. Things like stress, sleep, and "how" you approach your fitness goals are all "non-metabolic," yet nonetheless they *will* affect metabolism.

In the second part of this book, Scott discusses a lot of industry trends and scams as they relate to metabolism, while also providing a few alternatives. He talks about what "low carb dieting" really is, and what it really started out as, and why its current form is both silly and based on fear, rather than any being based on any truths about metabolism. He talks about Paleo dieting, what your protein needs are, and the truth about things like potatoes and coffee. (Namely, that it is ridiculous that many dieters are "afraid" of either of them.)

You shouldn't be afraid of food. You shouldn't have to count calories or worry that the 5 calories of ketchup you ate but forgot to track in your Excel spreadsheet will be the difference between success and failure. Obsessing about diet never leads anywhere positive.

Scott is absolutely "for" embracing structure and regimentation in your personal diet strategy, but that's because it means embracing routine and ritual, and ultimately *not* having to think about food all the time.

Human beings have had healthy metabolisms for millennia. It was not until after we started things like calorie counting and nutrient timing that things got screwed up, and for Scott, that's not a coincidence. But there's good news in that: it means that the way you keep a metabolism robust and healthy is relatively simple, and most of the strategies Scott mentions are things you can start doing today.

PART 1
What You Need To Know To Lose Weight

...And KEEP It Off!

Chapter 1.
A Calorie Is Not A Calorie

For decades, the calories in/calories out equation has ruled, but in the total context of weight loss (and real life) science has been calling that into question for years now, especially if we look at things longterm. The current nutritional and fitness-industry "math" simply doesn't add up.

Metabolically speaking, and looking at the bigger picture, a calorie is not a calorie.

Instead, what "really" matters, is the *metabolic* and *hormonal* environment of the body within which calories enter.

That's what determines how your body will deal with those calories. It's very easy to say, "Oh, based on this formula, your body burns 2,082 calories per day, therefore eat 1,582 calories per day to create a deficit of exactly 500 calories each day, to therefore create a total deficit of 3,500 calories per week, so that you lose precisely 1 lb each week."

When is weight loss ever that linear? The answer is never. Let's get real here, folks. Math like that never works out the way it should, does it?

The fact is the content of the calories you ingest will affect your hormones and your metabolism, which will in turn affect the number of calories you burn each day. You can't "out-calculate" your metabolism, because it's too complicated, too dynamic.

The complexity and truth of human metabolism explains why vogue industry trends like "IIFYM" (If It Fits Your Macros) or "IF" (Intermittent Fasting) can be terrible ideas for a majority of the people who follow them.

Look, I cite "The Twinkie Diet" all the time in my books. This is the case of Dr. Mark Haub losing 27 lbs by eating roughly 1,800 calories each day of Oreos, Twinkies, and other gas station foods, with a protein shake and a multivitamin. *Yes*, you can lose weight with those foods. *Yes*, Dr. Haub's work absolutely called into question our so-called "nutritional knowledge" and our whole approach to dieting. But the key takeaway from his work should not be, "As long as you count your total calories, you should eat whatever you want." The key takeaways aren't really metabolic. They have to do with mindset and how we think about and approach food and dieting. Because he was in a relative deficit, Dr. Haub didn't feel "deprived" while he was on his diet, and that is hugely important. He didn't choose some fashionable "eat this, not that" miracle diet. He simply created a slight deficit and went with it.

There are too many factors to consider for "calories in/calories out" to be the most relevant thing you consider in your weight loss goals. You need to consider the effects of those calories on hormones, their effects on longterm hunger and satiety, your body's metabolic compensation system, and more.

To reiterate:

<p align="center">The hormonal and metabolic environment of the body within which calories enter determines how your body deals with those calories.</p>

And to go along with that, your hormonal and metabolic environment doesn't just "reset" every 24 hours. The calories you ate yesterday will affect the hormonal and metabolic environment of the body into which calories enter today. In turn, the calories you eat *today* will likewise affect the hormonal and metabolic environment of your body *tomorrow*, when you'll need to eat more calories. Over time, these metabolic and hormonal effects will add up. There are not just immediate effects to the calories you ingest: there are residual and cumulative ones.

Even looking at those shorter term effects, 100 calories of M&Ms will be digested and assimilated and cause metabolic and hormonal responses that are much different than the ones caused by 100 calories of asparagus. Most people understand this at a gut level, yet still, dozens and dozens of frustrated people come to me for "diet solutions" each year after trying things like IIFYM. If that sounds like you, and you've been frustrated by the calorie equation not "adding up," you are not alone.

How many starts and stops and short-term "results" with long-term "consequences" are you going to experience before you ask what is wrong with the calorie equation itself, instead of thinking something is wrong with you for not "sticking to the diet," or blaming yourself for being "weak" when the weight inevitably starts coming back?

As Dan John once put it:

"The diet worked so well I had to quit following it."

Isn't this the common dieter experience?

Cutting calories too much and/or for too long makes you hungry and miserable and mentally preoccupied with food. When you stop the diet you will be metabolically primed to put the weight back on, for a myriad of biological and metabolic reasons.

As the old saying goes: money, food and sex all only really matter when you *ain't getting any*.

When it comes to the latter two in particular, food and sex, our brains have evolved to be extremely preoccupied with these things when we aren't getting enough. These are survival instincts. You can't skirt around a survival instinct for very long. After spending "12 weeks" or whatever it may be on some special diet, neurotransmitters in your brain will be screaming at you to *eat eat eat!*

Not only that, but over time, the caloric restriction will lead to less overall energy burning because a few things happen:

1) You aren't able to put in the same level of effort in exercise (weight training, sports, etc.) simply because you are too energy depleted.

2) Your body compensates for long-term calorie restriction by preserving energy in any way it can, something we call metabolic down-regulation.

3) Sports and training aside, you find you have less energy to do other things that used to burn calories and stoke metabolism as well.

We witness this in bodybuilding and physique competitors all the time (especially female physique competitors) who have no energy for anything outside the gym anymore. Daily tasks become "burdens," and this often includes even talking and thinking.

But hey, you're getting leaner "for now," so none of that matters… for now. Right?

Some people will also have more sensitive metabolisms that are more affected by these kinds of things. They might increase their physical activity to burn calories, but for them, due to their metabolic sensitivity, any increase in physical activity creates more hunger than it would in someone else, and eventually this leads to an increased caloric intake to compensate for that hunger. So they are healthy and more "physically fit," but their weight-loss stalls — this doesn't make them "weak." Their metabolism is different, more sensitive, and more ready to compensate against caloric restriction and dieting by increasing those hunger signals, or down-regulating its calorie burning, or both.

If you decrease your dietary caloric intake by a substantial amount while constantly increasing physical activity for the sake of burning calories, you'll find that it's an especially unpleasant experience—and not just for you, the dieter, but for anyone around you as well. You'll get short-tempered, tired, lethargic and it won't be pleasant for anyone. When I used to focus mostly on competitors in my coaching, as a contest got closer I wouldn't just ask *them* how they were doing... I would make it a point to ask their *spouses*. I often got exasperated "rolled eyes" as a response.

Some people are impressed by the level of effort and monumental willpower involved in that kind of sacrifice, but these bystanders seldom witness the fallout and consequences (for example, losing friends or upsetting loved ones because your diet has made you irritable and tired). It's especially easy to be impressed when you only witness the cosmetic results: a few before and after pictures, or what a dieter chooses to actually put on Facebook—say, a few nice photos and some inspiring quotes, but nothing about the mental turmoil, insane hunger, or relationship woes that their dieting has led to.

A long-term deprivation diet with no relief will generate intense hunger, and that will have all kinds of fallout and longterm consequences: physically, mentally, emotionally, and metabolically.

In worst case scenarios you'll get stalled or burnt out metabolisms, hormonal consequences, loss of muscle mass and other effects we now call "metabolic damage."

So… when ARE all calories equal?

Answer:

NEVER!

Your internal hormonal, biochemical, and metabolic environments need to be considered *first* and *foremost*. Sure, all calories are equal if you ignore all of the above, and you just choose not to think about how the body will react to those calories, but let's get real, folks.

There are thousands of people every year who experience short-term diet results only to suffer long-term consequences, yet after things have gone south, they don't understand that the short-term weight loss, and how they went about it, is what *caused* the long-term consequences. So what do they do? They try again, and things just get worse, because they're not addressing what actually matters. They're caught in the classic yo-yo dieting loop.

Remember that the body is quick to protect itself from attempts at absolute calorie deprivation. Many former dieters will tell you that they now "gain weight" even when eating healthy whole foods, and being very careful about what they eat.

How can that be?

It "be" because a calorie is not a calorie. The hormonal and metabolic environments in which calories enter are what matters!

You can damage and destroy that metabolic and hormonal environment when you put weight-loss ahead of metabolic support and optimization… *or* you can train your body to have a cooperative metabolism and healthy and productive hormonal environment.

Which one would you pick?

Chapter 2.
Calorie Math

One of my favourite expressions, with respect to this topic, is this:

"Calories do not measure metabolism."

"Metabolism," as such, is much more complex. It changes; it can be damaged; it can be made healthier or less healthy. The food you take in will affect it. Calories, by themselves, do not (accurately) measure metabolism, and that's why "calorie math" just doesn't work, practically speaking.

The real definition of a "calorie" is this:

"The amount of energy required to raise the temperature of a gram of water by 1 °C."

That's it, that's all.

A calorie is just a unit of energy. This has nothing to do with measuring the complex set of processes that make up human metabolism.

Calorie-counting cannot predict how foods with the same number of calories are going to act metabolically and hormonally in the body. Calorie counting also cannot predict how the body's current metabolic and hormonal environment will act on those foods.

While some very basic calorie math may be a fair *starting* place for a diet-strategy, it should definitely *end* there as well. It can be a general "reference point," but that's it.

I've used calories counts in several of my projects, but I used them because that is what people respond to and understand. I'm actually always hesitant to do so, because people tend to overemphasize the importance of the numbers when it comes to understanding the biology of weight-control.

The fitness and diet-industries lead people to obsess over calorie numbers – numbers that don't matter much in the grand scheme of things.

Many sites now have "calorie calculators" to "help" you with your fitness goals. Again, as a convenient *starting point* for Joe the First-Time Dieter, maybe that's fine. Most people aren't aware of how many calories are in this or that ingredient, or in this or that food, and having that information available can be convenient.

The problem is that an over-reliance on calculators and numbers leads to mental and emotional obsession.

I've witnessed it over and over again: someone begins by being "diligent" with tracking their exact calories. But that diligence soon becomes obsessive. Eventually that person is obsessed with tracking each and every calorie (which is impossible, since neither online databases nor nutrition labels provide near that level of accuracy), and before they realize what has happened, they have what is effectively an eating disorder.

The Current State of Health and Fitness

Sadly, things are not getting better. If anything, the fitness and diet industries are emphasizing "numbers" more and more. (This is partly due to the influence of the tech industry, of course—the whole idea of the "Quantified Self" and such.)

It's endless nonsense about numbers. Now we track:

- How many calories we eat.
- How many steps we take.
- How many calories we supposedly burn with 11 minutes on the elliptical, and then 16 minutes on the rowing machine, and then 10 more minutes on the...
- And on and on it goes...

Eating to live was never meant to be calculated like some kind of daily math equation.

People have been led to believe that they can "calculate their way thin." When things don't succeed, the fitness industry would have us believe that the problem is we're not doing *enough* weighing, measuring and counting!

What if that isn't even remotely true?

I've been lean for decades and I haven't counted calories in decades either. These things are connected, and have little to do with luck or coincidence.

I also take Sunday completely off from my diet-strategy... as this "day off" my diet strategy is actually a working part of my *overall* diet-strategy. On Sunday, I eat whatever I want to eat, and as much as I want to eat. When you factor in those Sundays, and you actually look at and "add up" the calories I eat, I should have been gaining weight incrementally all these years. Yet I haven't been. Why?

The answer is, as I said at the beginning of this chapter, because calories do not measure metabolism.

Humans were much healthier and slimmer a few generations ago, when most people hadn't even *heard* of calories or calorie counting. (Never mind being obsessed with it.) That's not a coincidence. The truth is that something *else* is disrupting and breaking our metabolisms — namely, the modern environment in which we live.

Complex calorie math is not a way out this disruption. It is an *illusion* of a way out, and an *illusion of control*. Often it is just one more thing to stress about (i.e. one more thing that can put your stress hormones into overdrive).

Let's address the faulty math. Calorie math simply doesn't add up, while biology does.

Here's one example:

Here's one example, taken from Chapter 1 Jonathan Bailor's *The Calorie Myth*. (Bailor puts the actual math bit in a footnote, but see the section called "Complexity Comes from Misinformation.")

In 2011 doctors at the University of North Carolina at Chapel Hill showed that the number of calories consumed per person per day increased by almost *600 calories per day* in the years between 1977 and 2006 (the actual average number was 570 cals per day, per person).

If calorie math was even remotely an accurate predictor of bodyweight and metabolism, then the "average person" who has increased their calorie intake by 570 calories per day between 1977 to 2006 should have also gained a massive amount of weight. To quote Bailor's calculations (in his footnote):

> "570 calories per person per day times 365 days in a year equals 208,050 calories. Multiply this by 8 years and we end up with 1,664,400 excess calories per person between 2006 and 2014. Divide 1,664,400 by the 3,500 calories in a point of fat and we get 476 pounds of fat per person."

To suggest that we are burning these extra calories off through activity is obviously ludicrous. To avoid the 75475 extra pounds of weight through exercise would require the equivalent of jogging for over 90 minutes every single day, 7 days per week, 365 days a year, for each day of those same 8 years. That's enough mileage to jog across the entire United States 11 times over.

None of these calculations take into account the changes in metabolism brought about by the extra calories, or by the extra weight, or by lifestyle changes (which would partly be totally separate from the increased calorie intake, but also partly a *result* of the extra calories and extra weight), or changes in metabolism brought about by the content of those calories.

As calorie-counting cultists love to point out: your metabolism is subject to the laws of thermodynamics. That means you won't gain weight eating 1,800 calories per day if you consistently burn just 1,801 calories per day. The laws of physics outright prevent this. Well, duh. But let's get real: that *massively* over-simplifies the metabolic processes. You won't "consistently" burn 1,801 calories per day.

With metabolism, there is always a complex interplay between the food you take in, your digestion, your metabolism, your energy needs, and the energy you draw from those calories, and how they make you feel (which affects energy, satiety, and on and on).

To put it bluntly: sustainable, realistic and longterm weight loss needs to address the *biology* of weight loss, not the "mathematics" of it.

Chapter 3.
The Metabolic Compensation System

In my discussion of why a calorie is not a calorie, I alluded to the importance of considering both the short-term and long-term consequences of what you eat.

As an extreme example, eating 900 calories of a few bits of lean chicken and then a bunch of leafy greens (as many physique competitors basically eat, because they're told to do so by irresponsible coaches) is going to result in serious hormonal consequences, not to mention a number of embarrassing gastric consequences as well.

When you're considering the biology of weight-control, you have to consider not just how calories themselves "add up," but how metabolic and hormonal effects "add up."

With that in mind, it is important to understand something called **"the metabolic compensation system."**

You can breakdown the effects into three different time periods:

1) The immediate effects

2) The residual effects

3) The cumulative effects

Keep that in mind when considering that weight-loss and sustainable weight-control play out over a long period of time, and that a diet is not just about "the now."

1. The Immediate Effects

Tell me if you've experienced something like this:

You decide to lose some weight, so you go on a diet, and you get into counting calories and proportioning your macros and all the rest of it.

These first few weeks of your diet, feel.... *marvelous*. Surprisingly so! You feel amazing. You wonder why you waited so long! You actually aren't extraordinarily hungry, and the weight seems to be melting off. You think you can do this forever. It's really not that hard, you feel great, it's working, and hey, what more could you ask for from a diet?

This is known as **"the anti-catabolic phase"** of metabolic compensation. (Anti-catabolic simply means the prevention of break-down of body tissues.) In the short-term, your body doesn't know that the lack of incoming food energy is going to take place over the long-term. Your metabolism burns off stored fat for its energy needs, so you lose weight.

But then things — frustratingly — go south. Why?

As you can probably guess, and as I said above, this is because there are three general phases of time to consider when discussing the metabolic compensation system:

1) The immediate

2) The residual

3) The cumulative

The mistake most yo-yo dieters make is to think all the positive responses to dieting that take place within the **immediate** realm of time are going to last forever, and that when they don't last forever, it's "their fault" or their "weakness" or something. That is untrue.

The immediate effects are simple the ones that most people associate with their dieting efforts. But the residual and cumulative effects are also a very direct result of those same dieting efforts, even if sometimes you don't experience or notice them until "after" the diet is over. (Sometimes you truly notice them for the first time the very specific "moment" the diet is over: that is, when the increased hunger and satiety causes that final cheat or binge that ends the diet.)

2. The Residual Effects

The metabolic compensation system is extremely adaptive, and this is even more true when considering the **residual** and **cumulative** effects of dieting, and any general lack of incoming food energy.

Here is what happens *after* those first few to several weeks of diet by calories-counting deprivation.

In the residual realm of time, your body makes its way into starvation mode. The human body knows no physiological difference between "a diet" and "starvation." Those labels are socially-constructed distinctions. Biologically, there is simply a large lack of energy.

How does a metabolism compensate and respond over time to less energy coming in than it requires for optimum function? It compensates by slowing down the rate of fat burning, and turning on its capacity for fat storing, because the body isn't stupid: it knows it needs as much stored energy as it can get, because for whatever reason, energy sources are becoming increasingly rare. It doesn't know this diet or perceived starvation won't go on forever, so it does what it can to prepare for that.

Most people have experienced an initial weight-loss on a diet only to have that weight-loss slow down, and slow down, then finally stall completely, even when eating what you would assume is a huge caloric deficit. This is due to your body adapting and "compensating" for the ongoing lack of caloric energy coming in.

Once the initial anti-catabolic phase of dieting is over, the body is no longer "tricked" by a lack of food energy. It responds to protect itself and survive. Instead of surrendering fat—as it did at the beginning—the metabolism now "compensates" by going into fat-*storing* mode to preserve as much energy as it can.

This metabolic compensation system also wants to shutdown any metabolically "expensive" bodily functions. This is often, for example, why women lose their periods as a diet wears on and they get leaner.

The metabolism also compensates by surrendering more and more metabolically active tissue to use as energy, instead of using fat. And what type of tissue is most metabolically active? Well, muscle tissue of course.

So in the "residual phase" of your diet, you may even likely still be losing weight, but *now you are losing the wrong kind of weight*. Bad news.

3. The Cumulative

Furthermore, as a result of this, as we move into the

"cumulative phase" of your diet, there will be metabolic hell to pay for surrendering lean muscle mass for energy needs, as the body simply keeps adjusting and compensating for the lack of adequate incoming food energy.

Lean muscle tissue is always calorically hungry. So when the metabolism realizes there is inadequate food energy coming in, your metabolism compensates by surrendering the calorie-hungry lean tissue (namely in the form of deamination, surrendering intramuscular BCAAs for use as energy) and it preserves its fat stores and even tries to store more of it. In other words, because of your ongoing diet via caloric deprivation, you have now turned on your fat-storing hormonal factory.

So the initial happy "anti-catabolic phase" of your diet that you thought was so wonderful kicked your metabolic compensation system into action, and eventually this lead to psychologically and biologically "unhappy" long-term consequences.

Here is more of what you need to know and embrace: even while you are in the immediate, anti-catabolic phase of dieting, eating less does not necessarily force the body to just burn bodyfat. Yes, there is an initial "anti-catabolic phase" where this is true. But this phase of the metabolic compensation system doesn't last very long.

How long this anti-catabolic phase is may be different for everyone. *But it always ends.* Eating less has one guaranteed long-term compensatory response from the body: if you eat less energy over a long period, you will burn less energy.

So let's review:

When human bodies need calories, and there aren't enough

coming in over the long-term, your internal metabolic and hormonal and biochemical systems (which are all connected) respond in several ways.

The most common response is to just slow the rate at which your body burns and uses calories, and to communicate to your body and mind that your body is tired and in need of more sustenance.

Simply slowing the rate of calorie burning is far easier for your body than it is for your body to convert calories from bodyfat to use as energy. Yes, that conversion will still go on to some degree, but slowing metabolism by using less and less stored energy (bodyfat) is the body's preferred response. After the short-term anti-catabolic phase of calories-restriction, the body's next preference is to tap into lean muscle tissue to use as energy.

This metabolic compensation response also sends a signal to thyroid, leptin and other hormonal systems, telling metabolism to slow down, use less energy, and raise hunger.

This is why so many contest-dieters get weaker and weaker as a diet wears on. In fact there is research that shows that, over the course of longterm caloric deprivation, up to **70%** of the weight lost (ignoring water weight lost) comes from burning muscle tissue, not fat.

When a diet process turns to muscle/lean tissue for energy, you might be losing weight on the scale, but you are setting off an emergency alarm inside your body.

Here's what will happen: You will get sick and tired of... well, of feeling sick and tired. You will be mentally, emotionally and physically exhausted by fighting constant hunger, and you will be ready to stop feeling terrible and irritable all day long. You will go back to eating a normal amount of food "just for now" (or so you tell yourself) but often this is when the floodgates open to binge eating, overeating and disordered eating and all the rest.

Or, you do indeed go back to eating just a "normal" amount of food and you stick to it, but even *then* your metabolism has down-regulated to burn less energy because of the long-term effects of your diet, and your hormonal systems and internal biochemical environment are now out of sync with each other in terms of healthy and balanced systemic function. (Out of sync in the sense that even when you're eating enough to gain back weight, the hunger signals *still* aren't winding down at all.) So even though you are eating a "normal" amount of calories again at this point and still feeling hungry, it is *like* "overeating" to your sluggish and down-regulated metabolism.

Moreover, because lean tissue sacrificed BCAAs for energy use, your body has also gone into "hoarding mode," so that it is hoarding incoming calories for fat storage, not using them to build of lean tissue (as it normally would with at least some of the excess calories).

Consider proof of all of this offered by George L. Thorpe, a physician working within *The American Medical Association*.

Way back in 1957 he explained in *The Journal of the American Medical Association* that eating less makes the body lose weight, yes, but, "Not by selective reduction of bodyfat only, but by wasting away of all body tissues as well." He says, "therefore, any success at weight-loss obtained by 'eating less' must be maintained by chronic under-nourishment."

And what happens when you keep a body chronically under-nourished? It gets sick and tired, doesn't it? It isn't practical or feasible to think you can continue to under-feed yourself and not experience the repercussions of that.

Yo-Yo dieting is the usual result. This throws your internal balancing mechanisms into complete chaos, and can make things worse. There is research that shows that the people who gain the most amount of unwanted weight in adulthood… are the ones who diet the most! Go figure.

Long-term weight-loss and sustainable weight-control is never about short-term diets. It is always going to be about creating a cooperative and optimized metabolic, hormonal, and internal biochemical well-functioning physiology.

So if you are considering trying another calories-counting/calories-restricted diet to lose weight, well two things come to mind 1) the oft-quoted definition of insanity and 2) wouldn't it just make better sense to heal and recover your metabolism, rather than struggling through life with a broken or damaged one?

Chapter References:

Keesey, RE and Powley, TL "The Regulation of Bodyweight" *Annual Review Psychology*, 1986, also see PubMed PMID 3963779

Leibel, RL et al, "Diminished Energy Requirements in Reduced-Weight Obese Patients" *Metabolism*. 1984

Thorpe, GL. "Treating Overweight Patients," *Journal of American Medical Association* 1957, see also PubMed PMID 8503353.

Young EA, et al "Hepatic Response to a Very-Low-Energy Diet and Refeeding in Rats" *American Journal of Clinical Nutrition*, 1993.

Chapter 4.
Metabolic Damage

No look at the biology of weight-control and metabolism would be complete without a discussion of metabolic *damage*.

I want to look at a very interesting research study on metabolism and the effects of dieting, done at The University of Geneva. Bailor also cites this one in *The Calorie Myth* (see the section titled "The Side Effects of Eating Less"). You can look at the references for more details. This study on diet and metabolism involved three groups of rats all eating the same quality of food.

1) **Group 1:** Were adult rats all eating normally

2) **Group 2:** Were adult rats temporarily losing weight by eating less

3) **Group 3:** Were younger rats who were "naturally" thinner and they weighed about as much as the rats from Group 2 after those Group

2 rats had dieted down and lost weight.

As Bailer points out, if this study were done on humans we could say that **Group 1**, the normal group, would be akin to a typical adult men or women around the age of 35. **Group 2**, the "eat less" group would be this same demographic of people who are now going on a diet, for their wedding or for some high school reunion or whatever; they are eating less calories and won't stop until they get to their goal weight or fit into a certain size of jeans from years ago. The **Group 3** rats, the naturally thin group, would be represented by people who are naturally slender and who have fit into their skinny jeans their whole lives without really ever dieting to do so. This makes for an interesting mix and comparison, doesn't it? Keep it in mind as we look at what the researchers found.

For the first 10 days of the research the Group 2 "eat less" group of rats ate 50% less than normal while the Group 1 "normal group" of rats continued to eat normally. This would be like comparing non-dieting adult people with folks doing diets like the HCG diet, the Bernstein diet and so on.

On the tenth day of the diet, Groups 1 and 3 kept eating normally and Group 2, the diet-by-deprivation rats, stopped the deprivation dieting and went back to eating normally as well.

But the research didn't stop at the end of the diet on the tenth day; instead, it went on for 35 days. This means that the Group 1 rats ate normally for 35 days; the Group 2 rats ate less than normal for 10 days, then ate normally for the next 25 days; and the Group 3 naturally thin group of rats at normally as well the whole time

So: at the end of the 35 days, what do you think the results of this study were in regards to changes in bodyweight, and in what direction?

At the end of the 35 days the Group 2 rats — i.e. the *only* group that dieted — weighed the most AND they had the highest bodyfat percentage!

Even though they only ate less than the other two groups of rats for 10 days – they were SIGNIFICANTLY heavier than the other two groups of rats who ate normally. Eating less for a sequence of time caused metabolic adjustments that led the Group 2 "dieting" rats to not just gain back what they lost during the first ten days, but to gain more as well!

This is what I refer to as "metabolic damage." Now, in place of rats, imagine the men and women I made comparisons to above. How many adult men and women do you know who go on "special diets" for some major event in their lives? Sure, the result is short-term weight-loss, but that is followed by long-term weight gain and fat gain!

The researchers in this particular study concluded that eating less – as in a deprivation diet – is actually worse than doing nothing at all.

Your body doesn't know the difference between diet and starvation. Those are psychological distinctions, not physiological ones. After a deprivation-diet the body's first priority is restoring all the bodyfat it surrendered on the diet. Its second priority is to protect itself in case that kind of starvation happens again.

Researchers have labeled this "bodyfat super compensation accumulation." Unfortunately, because weight gain is, for us human, and emotional issue, this bodyfat super compensation accumulation effect of dieting can also be a trigger for even further future weight problems, because when you gain back that fat, you'll no doubt want to diet again, and if you go about dieting in the same way, you start the cycle all over again… but it gets worse each time.

It's a cycle that is all too common. A person diets for the reasons outlined above. They lose weight for, say, a special event, and everyone comments on how great the look. Meanwhile, at the very same time, that person's body is building up defences against the weight loss. It is slowing its metabolism. Hunger and appetite centers are getting lit up. That person's short-term "successful" weight-loss turns into a long-term nightmare. They gain all the weight back, but they gain even more bodyfat as a percentage as well (because they lost a bit of muscle in the initial dieting, and they're primed for fat storing), just as with the rats above.

But now in the psychological realm (we aren't rats after all) that person feels embarrassed and ashamed. The solution? Well, this person reasons, they dieted once and lost all the weight, so they know they can do it again… they just have to do it "better and smarter this time." The just need "more willpower."

That is a lie that many dieters tell themselves, because

things are actually getting worse, not better.

So they go back on a diet and begin the cycle all over again. This is what the researchers mean when they say that the bodyfat supercompensation accumulation phase, or more simply, the "diet rebound," can be a trigger for future weight-gain and metabolic damage. This phase of metabolic adaptation is itself a trigger for another cycle of Yo-Yo dieting.

Researchers are now finding out something else I've been arguing for more than a decade now. When it comes to metabolic damage in the post-diet rebound period, you actually don't have to eat "a lot" in order to keep putting on weight.

The fact is, that just by going to back to eating "normally," like the dieting rats in this study, you can still gain a massive amount of weight very quickly. Even though these dieting rats were only eating the same amount of food as the Group 1 and Group 3 control group rats for the last 25 days of the study, they gained back a bunch of weight and *then some*.

Eating less slows metabolism, and when you feed a slowed, sluggish, or burned out metabolism "normal" amounts of food, and subject it to "normal" amounts of exercise, that person will gain more bodyfat.

The researchers in this excellent study illustrated that the Group 2 dieting rats' metabolisms were slowed by the dieting; they were burning bodyfat 500% less efficiently, and their metabolisms were correspondingly slowed down by 15 % by the end of the study.

Keep in mind these rats dieted *only* 10 days, yet the diet-rebound lasted at least two and half times that.

As a side note here, if you have the kind of metabolic damage I've described above, the worst thing you can do is "add cardio" to try to burn fat. To attempt to tap into the aerobic energy system when it is damaged this way is likely to further metabolic damage and hormonal disruption on several other fronts as well. For example, a metabolism slowed by 15% could easily become 20-25% if you add extra damage on top of it.

You may feel better by thinking you are at least "doing something" about the problem, but in the long-term you are likely making things worse for yourself, not better.

Researchers around the globe are now piecing together some of the damaging effects of prolonged calories-deprivation diets. But researchers are also looking at negative hormonal and internal biochemical consequences of dieting as well.

In the next chapter I'll look at another study that gives a bit more insight into metabolic damage.

Chapter References

Bailor, Jonathan *The Calories Myth*. New York: HarperWave, 2014.

Dulloo, Abdul G, and Lucien Girardier. "Adaptive Changes in Energy Expenditure During Refeeding Following Low-Calorie Intake: Evidence for a Specific Metabolic Component

Favoring Fat Storage." *The American Journal of Clinical Nutrition* 52 (1990): 415–420. Print. This above study is also discussed in Bailor's *The Calorie Myth* (Ch 4. See the section titled "The Side Effects of Eating Less")

Chapter 5.
More Research on Metabolic Damage

As I mentioned in the last chapter, the research is beginning to mount regarding "metabolic damage" as a result of dieting.

Here's another one Bailor cites in Chapter 4 (see "The Side Effects of Eating Less"). Consider this research conducted by Dr. Rudolph Leibel, director of the Division of Molecular Genetics at Columbia University Medical Center. He studied a group of subjects with an average weight of 335 lbs. who had used "extreme dieting" to get themselves down to an average weight of 220 lbs., achieving well over a 100 lbs weight-loss.

The research team wanted to study what effect this kind of dieting would have. They specifically wanted to study how the new, dieted-down 220 lbs bodies burned fat after this period of extreme caloric restriction. To do this properly, the researchers brought in two other control groups. One group was the same age as the 220 lbs. dieted-down group, but they were naturally slim, and weighed about 138 lbs. on average, without ever having really dieted to get there. The researchers *also* compared the dieted-down 220 lb group to a group of people *still at* 335 lbs. So, in essence this gave the researchers three groups to compare and contrast.

- **Group 1:** The *non*-dieted, original 335 lbs body weight subjects, before any dieting.

- **Group 2:** The "dieted-down" subjects weighed 220 lbs *after* losing 115 lbs.

- **Group 3:** The 138 lbs naturally slim subjects

What did the research show regarding the metabolic effects of extreme dieting to lose weight?

Recall that I have explained that during the short-term phase of any diet, the body goes through a brief "anti-catabolic phase" where it tends to surrender bodyfat easily, and it doesn't break down lean tissue. However, as time wears on during dieting, this short-term anti-catabolic effects of the diet don't last. Over the long-haul, the body burns lean tissue along with adipose tissue. This sends a direct message to the metabolic control centers of the body to sloooowwww down fat-burning and raise fat storing the moment the body gets the calories to do so.

The researchers wanted to know the metabolic effects

of extreme dieting: what were the energy needs and profiles of these dieted-down bodies compared to the control groups?

Before the study began, the non-dieting 335 lbs subjects required about 3,651 calories per day for basic metabolic functioning. They could eat that many calories, feel pretty good, and maintain their weight. Compare this to the control group of people weighing 138 lbs, who needed 2,280 calories per day for normal metabolic function. Now look at the dieted-down 220 lbs group: these people now needed only 2,171 calories to function. In other words, while dieting to lose weight, there was a *substantial* metabolic down regulation in these subjects. They still weighed 80 lbs *more* than their naturally slim counterparts, but needed *less* daily calories. In other words, the dieted-down group now must function on less incoming food energy than a control group that is 80 lbs lighter and smaller than them. (And that's after being "used to" consuming almost 1,500 calories more, each every day, back when they were still 335 lbs.)

How do you think this will work over the long-term?

This doesn't even account for the fact that the 220 lbs, dieted-down group is going to have increased hunger from the weight loss, so they would not only be hungrier than their 138 lb counterparts, they'd (presumably) also be hungrier than a 220 lbs counterpart who'd never lost any weight!

You can imagine how this can lead to problems as the body tries to "balance" and "correct" itself. This is not an isolated result; other researchers have drawn the same conclusions. It's not clear that their hunger levels would necessarily even be above 3,600 calories per day, such that even if they went back to eating what they ate before, they'd still feel unsatisfied, but it's not outside the realm of possibility, as you'll see below.

In my initial book on metabolic damage, I talk about the ground-breaking research of the now famous Ancel Keys study on "semi-starvation" (which, by the way, is hardly semi-starvation compared to some of weight loss diets I see, though it did go on for a fair while so that the effects could "add up" over time). I refer to Keys' Minnesota study often when explaining the physiological and psychological elements of metabolic damage over the course of long-term weight-loss and dieting.

In Keys' research, psychologically healthy and robust men were selected to go on a restricted diet of 1,600 cals per day for several months. The physiological, metabolic and psychological consequences to this "dieting" were unbelievable at the time. The subjects' metabolisms slowed down by a whopping 40%. Their strength level fell by 28%. Their endurance level fell by 79%, and perhaps most concerning of all, their **depression** levels rose by almost 40%.

And their hunger levels?

When the men in that study stopped eating less and the diet period was over and they were left to eat freely… *they averaged a whopping 5,000 cals per day*. They were *hungry*.

Does this sound like "optimum function" to you? Does that sound like hunger and metabolism are "in sync"? As we see in Liebel's research as well, these kinds of results are actually pretty normal, considering what the men went through.

How This Plays Out In The Real World

I call it "The Vacation Quandary."

A lady wants to drop some serious weight for her upcoming vacation. She goes on the HCG diet or some other silly diet that's making the rounds out there. So she goes on a restricted 500-800 calories regimen for 6-8 weeks before her vacation, and she of course begins losing weight. She's driven. She's diligent. She has a set date in mind, and real motivation to get there, and at first it's nothing but success. She's experiencing the *immediate* effects of dieting.

If you followed the two studies above, then you know there is a price to pay.

Before dieting, this woman, if she is of an average height of say 5'5" tall, and about 140 or 145 lbs, then she is likely needing about 2,000 cals per day or so to maintain that weight. But if her metabolism down-regulates by the same amount we saw in the studies above, she would end her diet needing something like only 1,200 cals per day (despite what any formulas for calculating calorie burning she finds online say).

When this person finally does stop eating less — partly because no one can sustain an absolute caloric-deficit, and partly because, hey, it's vacation time — she will introduce a normal amount of food (or more) to a metabolism that is no longer "normal." She "naturally" goes back to 2,000 calories per day or more, but her metabolism has now down-regulated to something like 1,200 calories per day. As well, her "fat storing capacity" has gone into overdrive, so not only is she is now gaining weight, she is gaining disproportionately more fat-weight relative to normal. (I.e., it's not lean muscle being added.)

Post-Diet Hunger and Fat-Storing Capacity

Remember that in the ground-breaking Ancel Keys Minnesota study I mentioned above, the men averaged 5,000 cals per day when they went back to eating freely.

Yes, they ate like that until they gained all their weight back and then some.

But here's the thing: *their lean tissue-to-fat proportions changed as it came back on.* After their post-diet weight-gain, their bodyfat percentage was now 52% higher on average than it had been before.

In short, all the lean tissue they surrendered on the diet was replaced by bodyfat, as their bodies went into what is now being called the "bodyfat supercompensation accumulation" phase of the post-diet rebound.

Keep in mind the Ancel Keys' research was done way back in 1950. Since then more and more research continues to reinforce the reality of this kind of "metabolic damage" from dieting too hard for too long.

Clearly, the conclusion that must be drawn here is that

the greater the degree of calories-deprivation the worse will be the inevitable rebound.

Even in my own Cycle Diet, I talk about the importance of two things:

- Using a **relative** calorie deficit, and NOT an **absolute** calorie deficit. (A relative calorie deficit is a minor calorie deficit *relative* to they person's normal requirements; an *absolute* deficit is something insane, like 600-800 calories per day, or even a bit higher.)

- Even if using a relative deficit, also implementing well-timed "refeeds" (cheat meals, cheat days, short-term diet breaks, and so on) of a substantial number of calories to prevent metabolic down-regulation and to optimize metabolism and hormonal and internal biochemical "co-operation" when trying to lean down.

What's the takeaway here?

Here is a simple phrase that encapsulates an entire philosophy of weight loss and physique transformation that will help *prevent* the above problems, *and* help deal with them:

"Force the body and it reacts; coax the body, and it responds."

We want the body to *respond* to our coaxing. Force the body with an extreme diet and it will only react against you. Coax it properly, though, and you can work *with* it towards your goals.

Extreme diets, or low calorie diets without appropriate re-feeds, lead to long-term metabolic consequences, yo-yo dieting, and a host of psychological disorders as well.

In the short-term, research has linked calorie-deprivation diets to:

- Lack of energy
- A compromised immune system
- A compromised reproductive cycle in women
- Adult ADD/ADHD
- Impaired cognitive function
- Irritability
- Low libido
- Disrupted sleep patterns

As researchers David Garner and Susan Wooley put it:

"It is only the rate of weight regain, not the fact of weight regain, that appears open to debate" (p. 740).

Let's not forget that these effect accumulate over time

when you factor in multiple bouts of dieting and weight regain.

A study done at The University of Pennsylvania took a look at this by getting rats to yo-yo diet. The rats dieted down in weight, then back up in weight, then again down in weight, then back up one last time. The second time that the rats tried to lose weight by eating less they lost weight at *half* the rate they did previously, and after the second diet they regained their weight 300% faster. The rats also stored bodyfat 400% more efficiently than the control rats who stayed on a consistent diet intake. (See Brownell.)

Part of my point is this: looking at diet and weight-loss in only short-term windows of time in the way that the fitness industry does — like 12 weeks transformation contests and so on — can cause severe long-term real-world weight issues down the road. If you're not thinking about the residual and cumulative effects of dieting, you're missing a substantial portion of the whole picture.

Consistency and coaxing are what it's all about. Don't be in it for that vacation that's coming up. Be in it for the long term; be in it for a long, healthy, happy life. A little vanity is perfectly okay, but realistically, you're actually doing your vanity no favours with a short-term diet that just causes weight-regain long term. You're much better off with a consistent, reasonable diet that coaxes your body where you want it to go.

Chapter References

Bailor, Jonathan *The Calories Myth*. New York: HarperWave, 2014.

Blackburn, GL, et al "Weight Cycling: The Experience of Human Dieters" *American Journal of Clinical Nutrition*, 1989

Brownell, Kelly D et al. "The Effects of Repeated Cycles of Weight Loss and Regain in Rats." *Physiology & Behavior* 38 (1986): 459–464.

Garner, David M, and Susan C Wooley. "Confronting the Failure of Behavioral and Dietary Treatments for Obesity." *Clinical Psychology Review* 11 (1991): 729–780.

Garrow, J S. "The Safety of Dieting." *Proceedings of the Nutrition Society* (1991): 493–499. Web.

Keesey, RE and Powley, TL "The Regulation of Bodyweight" *Annual Psychology Review*, 1986

Keys, A., Brozek, J., Henschel, A., Mickleson, O., and Taylor, H.L. *The Biology of Human Starvation* (2 vols) (1950) Minnesota: University of Minnesota Press

Leibel, Rudolph L, and Jules Hirsch. "Diminished Energy Requirements in Reduced-Obese Patients." *Metabolism* 33.2 (1984): 164–170. Print.

Chapter 6.
Restoring and Repairing a Damaged Metabolism

Every time I write an article about metabolic damage I get people contacting me with comments like, "So… what is the solution?"

People are looking to me for simple recipes for metabolic health and restoration.

Understand this folks: there is simply no such thing.

I realize that metabolic damage has now become an industry "buzzword" and unscrupulous wannabe gurus are trying to exploit the issue by promising you they have a one-size-fits-all answer. But as a real expert in metabolic damage, metabolic dysregulation, dysfunction and obstruction, I can tell you honestly this:

- **Everyone is different in terms of the degree of**

> metabolic damage and hormonal obstruction done to their bodies.

- Moreover, **everyone is different in terms of individual metabolic "resilience" in <u>counteracting</u> these issues and restoring metabolic health and hormonal balance.** What works for one person *may not ever work for another*, or may not work not nearly as well. You have to find what will work for you.

A broken bone takes time to heal, and the more severe the break, the longer will be the healing process. Radiation and chemotherapy may work for some cancer patients, but not for others. Bodies are unique.

Metabolic healing and restoration works on these same principles as well.

In this chapter I will address what the major indicators are in terms of the severity of metabolic damage and what it means in terms of possible healing, recovery and healthy restoration.

First, let's just get real about getting real. As the word "damage" implies, there is real fallout and collateral consequences that need to be considered. You can't just assume that, "Oh, it's broken... there must be an easy and simple way to fix it and be on my way." We need to stop that nonsense. Again, think of the broken bone example. You don't just head to the doctor, snap it back in place, and off you go back to everyday training; instead, you spend some time in a cast to let things heal and mend properly.

I am going to list some of the many factors in bullet-point form for your consideration. The more of these bullet-points you relate to and think "That's me!" the more severe your metabolic disruption and dysfunction and hormonal imbalance, and this means the longer and harder will be your way back to restoration, repair, and healing.

Factors Affecting Metabolic Damage

- How many years have you **Yo-Yo dieted**, gaining and losing, losing and gaining? (If you call this "competition-dieting," that doesn't change the metabolic reality that it is still yo-yoing in bodyweight. The body doesn't know the difference.) The more years you've dieted and lost, dieted and lost, then rebounded and then lost weight again and again – the more severe the damage is.

- Next: what is your **age**? Metabolism gets less and less resilient as you age, even for healthy metabolic profiles. Add metabolic damage/dysfunction and hormonal obstruction to this, and the more severe the damage is, and therefore the longer it will take to heal and recover and restore, if at all. If you are over 40, the way back gets tougher and tougher. That is the simple reality of it. It's not impossible, but it's certainly not easy.

- Next is **gender**. Estrogen likes fat and depends on it and vice versa. Mess with this with dieting again and again and women, relative to men, will have more metabolic dysregulation, dysfunction and hormonal obstruction as a result of repeated dieting.

- Next: **how healthy are you in general?** The more issues of ill-health you have along with metabolic damage then the harder metabolism will be to restore and heal.

- What is your **genetic** background? Like it or not, if your family and extended family are "big-boned" (translation: "over-weight") and you do damage to your metabolism and hormonal profile from repeated dieting, then the more severe the damage likely is as well.

- Next is **lifestyle**: "how" you live matters. If you are sleep deprived and prone to stress and anxiety this all just pushes you further and deeper into metabolic damage, metabolic dysregulation and dysfunction. **This one at least, you still have some control over. Take advantage of that!**

- Next is **prescription** meds. Even oral birth control in a hormonally and metabolically compromised system can make metabolic and hormonal healing more difficult. The more meds you take of the psychotropic variety (various anti-depressants, anti-anxiety meds etc.) the more severe your metabolic and hormonal obstruction is likely to be, and the longer they may take to heal as well.

- Then there is also your **"honest and actual" nutrition** to consider as well. Very often metabolic damage and the hormonal obstruction that goes along with it produce collateral damage in the guise of emotional suffering. People will begin to abuse food to find relief from emotional angst. Overeating, disordered-eating, binge-eating and just reaching for "convenient" but processed foods–these all take a metabolic and hormonal toll on an already metabolically compromised body as well. This can make the damage more severe and the healing and recovery time even longer as well. It does no good during this time to tell yourself, or to tell someone trying to help you to heal and recover your metabolism back, that you are "eating healthy whole foods all the time" when you really are not. The more disrupted and corrupted your healthy nutritional profile is, the longer metabolic healing and recovery will take as well.

- Next is **vitamin and supplement consumption**. Pay attention here! This is one area where observation and experience are ahead of the research. In a metabolically damaged and hormonally compromised and obstructed physiology, taking vitamins makes things *worse*, not better. For those of you trying to "supplement your way back to health" you are likely making the damage more severe and insidious and prolonging the time it will take to heal and recover, if at all. Nonsensical "cleanses" make things worse for you longer-term as well.

These above considerations paint a broad-outline of the factors involved in assessing the severity of metabolic damage and then creating a long-term plan for healing, recovery and restoration.

There is a lot more to consider here than just the "magic diet" side of the equation. There are exercise factors to consider as well and emotional fitness parameters to outline too.

Below I'll get into what the relevant research suggests regarding the exercise part of the equation when considering long-term metabolic healing. I know I sound like a broken record saying that there are no short-term solutions, but it is true. For something like this, you have to prepare yourself to deal with this honestly and in the long term. Trying to diet off 20 lbs because it is just so unsightly is, unfortunately, thinking in the short term. We have to get real.

Relevant Exercise Research

So, what are some things we *can* do? Thankfully, there is research on this we can use.

MD and PhD molecular cardiologist Y. Izumiya

showed that Type-2 muscle fiber stimulation in training can helped regress obesity and resolve metabolic and hormonal disorders in the obese mice with which he conducted his research.

This is what we are looking for in terms of treating metabolic damage. Thankfully, in simpler terms, what this kind of research means is that traditional bodypart and bodybuilding training can actually go a long way in restoring metabolic and hormonal profiles back to "healthy" again.

Note, though, that Dr. Izumiya doesn't talk about "burning calories" or "working up a sweat" or "training to exhaustion."

What he does talk about and emphasize is resolving metabolic and hormonal disorders. It's all about long-term emphasis.

In his research Dr. Izumiya describes how Type 2B muscle fibers play a role in increasing insulin sensitivity in a positive way and improving leptin profiles as well. He makes a special note to say that **these positive effects occur despite a decrease in overall physical activity.**

Quality of exercise and consistency are more important than the number of calories you burn (say, like adding "extra" cardio to burn fat, which can do just more damage in a metabolically or hormonally compromised system).

What's interesting here is that Dr. Izumiya is a cardiologist. You would expect him to have a bias towards, well, "cardio"-oriented exercise. But that's not the case! His research showed him something else, something better, especially when it comes to correcting metabolic and hormonal dysfunction and obstruction.

My suggestion for people battling these metabolic and hormonal issues is actually my **Hardgainer Solution workout program**, because the workouts reflect Dr. Izumiya's research. (No, I didn't initially design the program specifically to restore metabolic and hormonal function, but it will indeed have that effect over time.)

Dr. Izumiya's work isn't the only research to extoll the benefits of engaging type 2B muscle fibres. Researchers at Boston University showed that once again, exercise that consistently engages these Type 2B muscle fibers (glycolytic, not necessarily ATP/CP) can have an important effect on metabolic and hormonal health and balance.

The researchers wrote that stimulating these muscles fibers in a proper training environment "has a previously unappreciated role in regulating whole-body metabolism." Healthy and balanced metabolic regulation is what metabolic restoration, healing, and repair is all about.

The important point for me is that this training doesn't need to be "hardcore" and exhausting. Instead, it just needs to be consistent.

Sleep

Finally, in the factors affecting metabolic damage I listed above, I mentioned disrupted sleep-patterns. Research is showing more and more often that regular sleep patterns go a long, long way to promoting health, and this includes metabolic health.

Disrupted sleep pattern, by contrast, create a negative feedback loop that is tough to fix. That is, hormonal obstruction and metabolic dysregulation can be what initially leads to sleep disruption (because the hormones and neurotransmitters that help induce sleep get all out of whack). The disruption in sleep in turn reinforces the hormonal obstruction. That releases more stress hormones into the body, which in turn exacerbates these issues all the more.

The solution isn't to "power through it," but to pay attention to it! "Powering through" something like, say, sleep disruption, really will just make things worse. You have to address the underlying cause.

As I said earlier, a broken bone takes time to heal, and you heal it by not putting any stress on it. The more severe the break, the longer the healing will take, and even then that is if the bone is "set and rested."

A broken metabolism works the same way. You can't heal it by putting more stress and strain on it, any more than more stress and strain on a broken bone can heal it.

"Going harder and longer" (to burn more calories) is not the solution to metabolic and hormonal dysfunction and obstruction caused by dieting. In fact "going harder and longer" is what likely gave you metabolic damage and hormonal obstruction in the first place. How is "more of the same" any kind of solution?

Similarly, eating less in order to lose rebound weight

will disrupt sleep, and that disrupted sleep will prevent metabolic and hormonal recovery, restoration and healing. It will result in further metabolic compensation. Things will get worse, and worse, and worse. At that point exercising more because "eating less" isn't working would be a fool's game. That is how you *stay broken*; it's not how you recover and heal!

Sleeping less or disrupted sleep patterns increases stress. Moreover, working out "to burn calories" when you already have a compromised metabolism is a lot like exercising a freshly broken bone to make it heal faster.

Add to that mix a "calorie-deprivation" diet in a compromised metabolism because "you want to lose weight" and you'll just keep inflicting more and more damage upon your body.

I know darn well I might sound like a broken record, but I'll say it again anyway: healing and recovery and restoration require "less stress," not more.

What is required is more honest attention to what you need, and less ego prioritizing of what you want. Fixing a broken metabolism requires *nurturing* it, not pounding it.

Chapter References

Bailor, Jonathan *The Calorie Myth*. New York: HarperWave, 2014.

Izumiya, Y. et al., "Fast/Glycolytic Muscle Fiber Growth Reduces Fat Mass and Improves Metabolic Parameters in Obese Mice," *Cellular Metabolism*,

2003.

Kolata, Gina. *Ultimate Fitness: The Quest for Truth About Exercise and Health.* New York: Farrar, Straus & Giroux, 2004.

Chapter 7.
Exercise I: Quality Over Quantity

Not all bodies are equal in terms healthy and natural metabolic and hormonal function.

Think of it like lining up at a starting line for a race. Many of you are going to be lined up 20 or 30 yards beyond the official starting line. Previous ill-advised dieting has likely created hormonal obstruction and dysfunction in you. Metabolically, ill-advised dieting might have created metabolic dysregulation, burnout, and a sluggish or down-regulated metabolism.

Remember that the **metabolic**, **hormonal**, and **internal biochemical** environments are the "Big Three" of weight-control, and they are meant to work in harmony and in synchrony with each other.

When one of these three is thrown out of whack, the other two usually follow, simply because of the body's many checks and back-up systems.

When dieting or "bad eating habits" throw one of these into disarray, and you find yourself in that position, then using exercise to correct it can become *more* problematic as well.

Exercise:
More Does <u>Not</u> Equal Better

When someone is overweight and trying to shed pounds permanently, "more" exercise is not better when it comes to resetting hormonal systems and getting your metabolism working correctly. In fact "more" exercise for overweight people, even fit overweight people, will often just make you tired, without there being any real added positive effects for hormones or metabolism.

Furthermore, more exercise for those of you who have thrown your metabolic and hormonal systems into disarray and dysfunction, will do more harm than good in you as well, when it comes to re-setting your system and making it right again.

For example let's look at a study on overweight women conducted by Timothy Church. In the study, Church worked with college-aged, overweight women and had them burn 2,000 cals per week through exercise for eighteen months. What happened? These women experienced NO weight-loss, even though they were burning 2,000 calories per week in exercise. (If you do the kind of calorie math we already know is rubbish, over 18 months, or 78 weeks, they should have lost an average of 44.5 lbs. Nope. Didn't happen. They lost *nothing*.)

Church divided the women into 4 different groups:

1) No change in exercise
2) Exercise more
3) Exercise even more
4) Exercise WAY more

He noted that "more exercise" in overweight subjects doesn't lead to more bodyfat being burned. In fact he concluded that a high dose of exercise for overweight people supports previous studies' findings that high amounts of exercise trigger "compensatory mechanisms" that "attenuate weight loss."

To put it bluntly: the calorie-burning focus of the way we often approach exercise is faulty. The focus of exercise needs to be on getting metabolic and hormonal systems back in sync with each other, and back into a healthy state. The means *quality*, or doing the right kind of exercise. *Quantity* is usually about just trying to "burn more calories," but that's not what will help.

When it comes to exercise, instead of a focus on calorie-burning, people with these issues should focus more on tissue-building exercises that will optimize and balance metabolic and hormonal function *over time*. Focusing on short-term windows of time can blind someone to the long-term consequences.

When it comes to course-correcting metabolism and

hormonal balance and function, the type of exercise matters as well. For overweight people who think "cardio" (as in aerobic training) is the answer, this can be a huge mistake.

In Timothy Caulfield's *The Cure for Everything*,, experienced marathon runner Kim Raine said this:

> *"I've run eighteen marathons and I put one pound <u>on</u> for each one. Eighteen marathons and eighteen pounds heavier. It is so maddening!"*

Yet this is a very common experience among women. A damaged and dysregulated metabolism will not be "set right" by adding aerobic work, or only doing aerobic work with that purpose in mind. The aerobic energy system simply doesn't seem to play a role in course-correcting metabolic and hormonal function and making it right again.

Furthermore, training to "lose weight" while pretending to be trying to course correct metabolic and hormonal function can be a lie you tell yourself. Just because you want weight-loss and a healthy reset metabolism and hormonal system to go together doesn't mean both these things will happen at the same time. Weight-loss cannot be the primary goal while working on course correcting metabolism and hormonal systems. The metabolism and hormonal systems need to come first.

Now, to be clear, it may certainly be that if someone is

not just overweight but obese then walking—just plain old "walking"—can be a healthy and viable exercise path to begin the process of resetting metabolism and hormonal systems. But for people overweight by say 30-60 lbs. or less, and people who have gained weight as a consequence of deprivation dieting, then walking, jogging, running and so on is not likely to do much of anything for fat burning and leanness over the long-term.

As a side note let me just add a quick word on "jogging" and running here. Misinformed fitness enthusiasts are often under the mistaken impression that these forms of exercise are "healthier" and "better" than other forms of exercise, and this is not necessarily true at all. What *is* true is that running and jogging cause more injuries than any other form of exercise, and create a mess when it comes to knee health and hip alignment, foot issues, and more. The American Heart Association, while usually on the side of "aerobic training," found that jogging injures more than half the people who take it up as a form of exercise activity. This is hardly a statistic that endorses this form of exercise. Imagine if your child wanted to take up some sport where more than the half the kids taking part in it got injured—would you let them?

The number of injuries you get are basically because for every mile you run, your feet hit the ground 900 times. Even if you only weigh 150 lbs. then you are thumping 135,000 pounds of force against the joints and ligaments, starting with the feet and extending into the knees, hips, low back and even the shoulders. As some exercise researchers have put it, "Jogging is healthy exercise for the body like boxing is healthy exercise for the head and face." Of course, there is big business in running shoes and all the rest, so there are ample reasons in dollars and cents for the widespread promotion of this form of activity and making it sound simple and safe, but for most people, running and jogging are terrible choices for long-term exercise.

Running and jogging are the only forms of activity you really should be "built for doing" and that build includes being light to begin with. For people with weight to lose, and for people with metabolic and hormonal obstruction and dysfunction set in motion by previous calorie-restriction dieting, you are by definition not build for doing it. In that case, such activity is simply not a wise exercise vehicle to get you to where you want to go, either in terms of weight-loss or to help you course-correct optimum metabolic and hormonal function.

For all the bashing traditional bodypart and bodybuilding training has been taking of late, it is still the superior form of exercise in course-correcting metabolic and hormonal and internal biochemical functions, and getting these systems back in sync with each other. This kind of training targets Type 2B muscle fibres, which, to make a long story short, will help with metabolism and hormonal function. Even better would be whole body training, or body part training done in complexes from supersets to trisets — what has been termed "strength-density" training. This is a very safe form of exercise, since it exercises muscles with resistance and through a fully-intended range of motion around a joint. It should be far less ballistic in nature as well. These workouts do not have to be "all out" efforts, either. In fact, monitoring oxygen debt so that breathing is slightly labored, yet doesn't reach the level of "panting," ensures adequate intra-workout recovery (recovery within a single workout) and this leads to inter-workout recovery (recovery between workouts) as well.

I am currently in the process of gathering more research into how to course-correct metabolic and hormonal function damaged by calorie-restriction dieting.

But honestly? The answer is easier and simpler than most people want to believe. The real issue is that it can be hard accept that the process takes longer than one would want it to. The temptation is to "do more" in order to burn more calories. But the research, and my own experience working with clients, show that this is a fool's game. If you have damaged your metabolic and hormonal regulating system because of dieting and working "on" your body, you have to accept that this can take time. You have to move away from working "on" your body, and start learning how to work "with" your body.

Chapter References

Bailor, Jonathan *The Calories Myth*. New York: HarperWave, 2014.

Caufield, Timothy. *The Cure for Everything: Untangling Twisted Messages about Health, Fitness, and Happiness.* Beacon Press, 2012.

Church, Timothy S et al. "Changes in Weight, Waist Circumference and Compensatory Responses with Different Doses of Exercise Among Sedentary, Overweight Postmenopausal Women." Ed. Thorkild I A Sorensen. *PLoS ONE* 4.2 (2009): e4515. Web.

Chapter 8.
Exercise II: How Cardio Can Make You Fat

In the last chapter I mentioned research that shows that if you suffer metabolic dysfunction and hormonal obstruction issues because of previous diets and weight-gain cycles, the kind of exercise that helps you back to restorative health is exercise that targets the Type 2B muscle fibers. This is the kind of training that is known as "bodypart" training, whether totally traditional or training through complexes (super sets, tri-sets, and so on). The exercise doesn't have to be intense or exhausting. In fact, that level of intensity may also keep you trapped in the metabolic damage and hormonal obstruction cycle.

However, since I still get many emails asking me about cardio, or questioning why or how cardio isn't that good for you, from people whom I *know* have read previous work saying "don't do cardio," this chapter is all about the reasons why cardio can keep you fat, and why it is *not* the answer. It's not as effective at calorie burning as you'd think, and too much cardio slows metabolism further.

Many people have been led to believe that if you add cardio in the form of aerobic exercise you are doing a good thing to restore your metabolism and burn off the rebound body-fat weight-gain. But in a metabolically dysfunctional and hormonally obstructed body this is patently NOT TRUE.

If you think you are doing aerobic training to "burn fat" or to "raise metabolism" that is simply not the case.

Look around your local gym environments in the months following some local Figure or Bikini contest. Who do you think rebounds the most in weight and fat gain after such a competition? The answer will always be the ones who did the most aerobic activity to get contest-ready. Always!

(If you're not involved in that world, know that figure and bikini competitors can often be told to do *hours* of cardio each and every day. As you can imagine, this is exhausting and horrible for metabolism, and the rebound is exactly as bad as you'd expect.)

Recently someone told me about training at a local fitness boot camp. There are pictures of two of the class leaders on the wall from when they competed in a physique competition. The person who'd gone to the boot camp emailed me and said, "The first instructor has gained *at least* 100 lbs compared to the picture on the wall! When I finally met the second group instructor, she'd gained at least 60 lbs since those pictures were taken! What is going on here? Who leans out like that and then gains 100 lbs after?" I told this person the truth: many competitors go through insane cycles of dieting and cardio to get lean, and then they have massive rebound weight-gain. It's become part of the culture, and nutrition and dieting coaches are still giving programs with that kind of insane cardio regimen built in.

Not only is aerobic training not the best exercise for fat loss, in a metabolically compromised body it can actually enhance fat storing. Think about that for a minute. Not only does aerobic exercise not raise or optimize metabolism, it can cause metabolism to further down-regulate. This effect is even more pronounced if dieting has put you in a metabolically dysregulated and compromised state. I deal with the fall-out of this every single day.

If you are doing a lot of "pre-contest" aerobic activity, or you are doing lots of cardio to "get lean and lose weight" you may be clinging to an out-dated and wrong-headed notion that may set you back, *way* back, even if it feels like you are "making progress" initially.

The dieting body responds to a lack of calories, combined with aerobic training, by slowing metabolism and signaling for more enhanced fat storage. With that in mind, would 12 weeks or so of dieting for some lame online "transformation contest" have any beneficial long-term metabolic or fat burning effects? Answer: *Heck* no.

We need to also get away from lame notions like

counting or "tracking" how many calories you think you are burning off during your cardio because some "machine" spits out a number. Resetting metabolism and restoring balanced hormonal function and health have little to do with burning off calories first.

Dr. Eric Oliver, in *Fat Politics*, citing the work of Dr. Roland Weinsier, gave the following estimates regarding the effectiveness of calorie burning through exercise:

> For Americans to begin losing weight through exercise, the current USDA exercise guidelines would have to be increased by almost 200 percent. In other words, Americans would need to start exercising at least two hours a day, six days a week for their weights to start going down. (Oliver p. 152)

Clearly exercise calorie burning is not the answer.

The answer is to stop the focus on calorie math when it comes to exercise, and to start focusing on exercise that supports and promotes healthy metabolic and hormonal profiles! There is indeed a "right" form of exercise for promoting and supporting healthy metabolism and hormonal function. As I said, the form of exercise to focus on is traditional bodybuilding approaches, more or less. Smart exercise is not about how many calories you burn, it's about optimizing metabolic and hormonal function, via a very specific kind of muscle-stimulation.

But make a note here as well: this has nothing to do with thinking you have to add 50 lbs. of muscle to your body in the process. Moreover, for any women afraid of lifting weights, let me tell you: it is simply not true that by lifting weights, you will "get huge." It's especially untrue for women, whose testosterone levels match that of a 10 years old boy. There aren't many huge and ripped 10 years old boys walking around out there.

It is a fact that "aerobic activity" triggers a cortisol response that is catabolic, not anabolic, to the tissue-building process. Aerobic activity has also been proven to suppress the anabolic hormones. For example, long distance runners suffer sustained and prolonged suppressed testosterone production.

The Aerobic Myth is still being perpetuated in gyms all across the world. When I travel, hotels that advertise having the "best gyms" always show their shiny expensive cardio equipment and seldom show their weight-training, or resistance-training equipment.

For a bit more proof on the ineffectiveness on cardio, take a look at some of the research.

Some of the research:

- Try this one in *The Journal of Sport Nutrition* (see Utter et al.). The findings were that 12 weeks of 45 minutes of aerobic training had no effect—yes absolutely *zero* effect—on body composition, relative to just dieting alone for the same period of time. That sure seems to be a tremendous waste of gym time over a three month period.

- In *The Journal of Clinical Endocrinology & Metabolism*

(see Redman et al.), this study asked what is the effect of diet plus aerobic training on body composition relative to diet alone? Findings were that 50 minutes of aerobic training performed 5 days per week over 6 months had *no additional effects on body composition*. More wasted time.

- In the journal *Obesity* (see McTiernan et al.), the hypothesis was this: "What are the exercise effects on weight and body fat in men and women?" This twelve-month study looked at six hours of aerobic training per week (one hour per day, six days per week), and the average weight loss was 0.5 lbs… *per month*.

- In *Metabolism* (see Tremblay et al.). Hypothesis: Does more calories burned during training yield more fat loss? This study looked at 20 weeks of endurance training vs. 15 weeks of interval training. The findings were that while the interval group burned less than half the calories *during* training, this group also showed a *nine times greater fat loss than the endurance group* over the course of the study. The number of calories being burned or not burned during exercise sessions doesn't matter.

- In the *Journal of American College of Nutrition* (see Bryner et al.). In this study, the aerobic group exercised four times weekly, and the resistance training group exercised three times weekly. VO2 Max increased in both groups, but the resistance training group lost "significantly" more fat and did not lose any lean body mass, even at 800 calories per day. Furthermore, the resistance training group actually increased metabolism. The aerobic training group lost lean body mass (so they looked a bit worse, *and* their metabolisms would have slowed as a result).

On the exercise side of the equation of repairing a metabolism, learning to work towards long-term healthy metabolic and hormonal effects means forgetting about a focus on cardio, or on calories burned *during* exercise, as well as letting go of "the aerobic myth" more generally.

In short, it means letting go of "quantity" of exercise and focusing on "quality" of exercise.

Chapter References

Bryner, Rand W et al. "Effects of Resistance vs. Aerobic Training Combined with an 800 Calorie Liquid Diet on Lean Body Mass and Resting Metabolic Rate." *Journal of the American College of Nutrition* 18.1 (1999): 115–121. Print.

McTiernan, Anne et al. "Exercise Effect on Weight and Body Fat in Men and Women." *Obesity* 15.6 (2007): 1496–1512. Print.

Oliver, J. Eric. *Fat Politics: The Real Story Behind America's Obesity Epidemic.* New York: Oxford UP, 2006.

Redman, Leanne M et al. "Effect of Calorie Restriction with or Without Exercise on Body Composition and Fat Distribution." *The Journal of Clinical Endocrinology & Metabolism* 92.3 (2007): 865–872. Web.

Utter, Alan C et al. "Influence of Diet and/or Exercise on Body Composition and Cardiorespitory Fitness in Obese Women." *International Journal of Sport Nutrition* (1998): 213–222. Print.

Tremblay, Angelo, Jean-Aimé Simoneau, and Claude Bouchard. "Impact of Exercise Intensity on Body Fatness and Skeletal Muscle Metabolism." *Metabolism* 43.7 (2003): 814–818. Print.

Chapter 9.
Dieting As You Get Older

For people who are 40 and over, and for perimenopausal women, you face a double-edged sword when it comes to weight-control. It is very likely that will you gain *some* unwanted weight during these years – but it is even more likely that severe calorie-deprivation dieting as an "answer" to such weight-gain will cause more harm than good.

As we age, out metabolisms become more sensitive, and we have to be more careful.

Our hormones change as we get older. This is true of everyone. If you add dieting into the mix, you can turn what is natural weight gain into an out-of-control spiral. Calorie-counting and calorie-deprivation are not the way out of weight-gain for you as you get older.

Consider this startling long-term study by Sumithran et al. published in *The New England Journal of Medicine*.

Fifty men and post-menopausal women forced themselves to eat less for 10 weeks. (If you can't tell, the keyword here is "forced.") To no one's surprise, they all lost weight... initially. What the study revealed is that forcing weight off creates dysfunction and obstruction in the hormonal and metabolic feedback loops that operate to control weight and to function in a healthy manner (e.g. peptide YY, cholecystokinin, gastric polypeptides, ghrelin, and leptin, just to name a few). This is what happens when you to try to override your biological hardwiring.

So what were the consequences to this disruption and obstruction, after the 10 weeks of dieting were over?

As a physiological response to the lack of energy coming in, the subjects' appetites and cravings increased. To go along with this, the number of calories they burned also decreased at the same time. As you can imagine, this is a terrible combination for long-term weight-control. Their internal biochemical and hormonal and metabolic systems were adjusting for the lack of energy coming in.

No one fools the body for long, and no one forces the body into change without it going into survival mode. The subjects' bodies were fighting back to return them to their previous bodyweight set point. The body does not know the difference between a calorie-deprivation "diet" and real starvation. The body will respond to both scenarios the same way—by protecting itself for survival. Anyone familiar with my writings about the consequences of dieting knows that the result seen in this study is not a novel or unusual outcome.

For the past few decades, there has actually been a fair bit of research about the biological, metabolic and hormonal adaptations to forced dieting (consider Ansel Keys' work in the 50s). But *this* study kept going where other studies usually stopped; this one really showed the long-term effects. These researchers showed that even one whole year after following a mere 10 weeks of forced calories-deprivation, the alterations in appetite, cravings, and slower calories-burn continued to persist, even a *year* after the dieting had stopped and the weight was regained!

What this research study showed is the body's instinctual desire to "fight back." And the body fights back long-term, as a sort of "biological insurance policy" if you will.

As for the older participants in this study, well, their biological, metabolic and hormonal systems were synergistically engaged for the longterm in multiple compensatory mechanisms, all to get the body to do everything it could do to restore itself to its previous set-point. Part of this includes implementing biological, hormonal, and metabolic safeguards to prevent that kind of weight-loss from happening again: your body makes you hungry, and makes you crave more food, because it wants you to store more food, just in case.

The researchers noted that the "changes in appetite persist[ed] for 12 months," and there was a "greater-than-predicted decline in 24-hour energy expenditure" (p. 1603). Even a year later, the subjects' bodies were still "vigorously resisting" this misguided attempt at weight-loss-thru-calories-deprivation, and their systems were "desperately trying to regain weight."

This is just one example of many.

If you really want long-term weight-loss and sustainable weight-control, you have to rethink the whole notion of the term "diet." **I prefer the term "diet-strategy," and such a strategy must always entail long-term considerations and the metabolic compensatory system as well.** This is the biology of weight-control and it must be considered and understood if your goal is substantial and sustainable weight-loss.

The key is to *coax* your bodyweight set-point down in a way where your body is not threatened. You have to learn to work *with* human biology, and not think you can force it to do anything other than what it has evolved to do. If you're older, that means factoring your age in. If you got away with hard dieting when you were younger, that is likely no longer the case.

What most people require now for long-term sustainable weight-loss and weight-control is not a laser-like focus on dieting and weight loss; rather, what's need is a focus on metabolic healing and recovery! This becomes especially true if you are over 40 and have weight to lose and/or if you are a peri-menopausal woman seeking to optimize metabolic and hormonal function in a way that supports fat loss while preserving lean mass.

You can't do that through the usual diet-mantra of calorie math. It's just not how your body works. Your body is even more susceptible to "metabolic dysregulation" as you age and try to diet off weight.

There is no secret "dieting as you get older" metabolism quick fix recipe I have, except to be more careful with dieting, and to re-iterate a lot of what I've already said in this book. What I've already said simply becomes more true as we age and our metabolisms becomes more sensitive and quicker to compensate against a deprivation diet. Now more than ever it is important that you work *with* your body, not against it!

Chapter References

Keys, A., Brozek, J., Henschel, A., Mickleson, O., and Taylor, H.L. *The Biology of Human Starvation* (2 vols.) (1950) Minnesota: University of Minnesota Press

Keesey, Richard E, and Matt D Hirvoven. "Body Weight Set-Points: Determination and Adjustment." *The Journal of Nutrition* 127.9 (1997): 1875S–1883S. Print.

Sumithran, Priya et al. "Long-Term Persistence of Hormonal Adaptations to Weight Loss." *The New England Journal of Medicine* 365.17 (2011): 1597–1604.

Chapter 10.
Stress and Metabolism

When you read online fitness blogs, or magazines, there is a very real tendency to separate all matters that influence "wellness." The idea of "fitness" is compartmentalized into matters of diet and training... and then not much else. If they are included, it's as an after thought: "Oh yeah, and make sure you get good sleep while you diet."

The fitness, diet and nutrition industries would have you believe that the mind is either independent of the body, or that the mind is influenced by the body, but never the other way around.

The mind and body are deeply interconnected, but this isn't a one-way street. It's a multi-laned, multi-directional highway. The mind is the brain's experience of itself. The brain is part of the body proper, and is composed of life tissue. To think there is "separation" between mind and body, or body and mind, is near-sighted and incomplete.

Because your mind is linked by brain to body and back again, things that affect the mind also affect all parts of the body and physiological function.

Studies are pretty clear that factors that lead to a state of mental well-being and happiness enhance physical health. Conversely, things that diminish your sense of well-being can cause actual physical sickness and other ill effects. It's very common for the overstressed, overworked, overscheduled adult to be the one who catches the most colds, flus, and whatever contagious bug is going around at the time.

These matters of immune system health do no "just" boil down to nutritional status, but the status of your stress levels as well.

Your health, and your metabolic health, are not *just* about diet, nutrition and exercise. As the saying goes: so often you look to remedies by examining what you are eating, when really, you need to examine what's eating you.

Chronic stress and all its forms, including "worry" are also damaging to physical health and can negatively impact metabolism. Also: worrying and stressing about your diet or the number on the weight scale is still a form of worrying, of anxiety and of chronic stress.

Episodic stress here and there is a part of life and will strengthen you, making it easier to be more emotionally resilient next time you are faced with challenging circumstances. But when these stressors are chronic and never let up, they will show in your body and on your body.

It is documented for instance that IBS (irritable bowel syndrome) responds "especially well" to placebo treatments, an indication that its causes are often emotional, not purely digestive. Similarly, autoimmune diseases are on the increase but so too on the increase are people's reported levels of "unmanageable stress." I doubt this is just coincidence, as prolonged, unmanageable stress has a known effect on the body's immune system. The mind affects the body just as much or more than the body affects the mind.

When you focus only on "nutritional" or "supplemental" solutions to feel better, or improve metabolism or lose weight or whatever, chances are you are looking in the wrong place and always will be.

If your job, your relationships, or your other life stressors consistently keep you up at night, and they keep you from getting high quality and adequate quantity of sleep... you can't "diet" your way out of this scenario, nor can you supplement your way out of it, nor can you "physically train" your way out of it.

Trying to start a new diet or exercise regiment may contribute to feeling better in some small way (the mind affects the body, after all), but in and of themselves they do not "remedy" the actual root issues of modern stress and how you experience it.

You either control and own your stress, or it controls

and owns you! If stress controls you, then you likely won't be able to lose those extra pounds anyway. Adding the goal of weight-loss or leanness to your "to do" list if you are already a person feeling lots of stress will merely add more and more stress to a life that already isn't dealing with stress in a healthy and empowering way to begin with.

A multi-vitamin or some anti-oxidant formula isn't going to suddenly give you enhanced mental and emotional and spiritual fitness. Just like exercise is required to enhance physical fitness, be healthy and control bodyfat, so too is mental and emotional exercise required to enhance mental fitness to control your stress.

Let's also be clear that physical fitness and physical appearance are two different things in this regard when it comes to "feeling and experiencing" wellness in an authentic way. This focus you might have on how you look can more often than not be upside down and backwards. Your body that you don't like – that is also a source of stress to you – but chances are it looks this way as a reflection of your inner self; weighed down by all the angst you haul around with you each day by avoiding your mental fitness, emotional fitness and spiritual fitness exercises.

We need to stop buying into cleverly designed industry notions that you can "feel better" simply by "eating this and not that" or by swallowing a pill from "supplement brand X."

The path to an optimized and coaxed metabolism begins with looking at the bigger picture. There is no secret metabolism boosting diet. You can have a very *good* diet that includes healthy whole foods, adequate protein sparing nutrients, and which creates just the right amount of "tolerable hunger" and so on. I'll talk about all that. But if you don't look at the bigger picture and consider things like sleep, work stress, relationship stress, and anything else that might "weigh you down," you will more often than not fail to get at the root causes.

If metabolism is, as I've argued, a dynamic and complex process that is much, much more than "calories in/calories out," then it absolutely includes things like sleep (or sleep deprivation), stress, happiness, unhappiness, and all sorts of other aspects of our lives that have nothing to do with you macro breakdown or the number of calories you eat each day.

Chapter 11.
Seven Magic Words For a Healthy Metabolism

If you've done a lot of reading about nutrition and eating, then at some point you have come across these fantastic seven words by journalist Michael Pollan:

"Eat food, not too much, mostly plants."

These simple seven words condense thousands and thousands of pages of nutritional texts into a comprehensive and viable diet-strategy for health, wellness, fitness and leanness… oh, and metabolic health.

Sometimes it takes a journalist to simplify what scientists and researchers continue to make more complicated. It can be easy to get side-tracked by the over-abundance of seemingly conflicting information that circulates in the media.

You run into arguments like the following:

- "Dairy is healthy" vs. "Dairy will make you sick"
- "Meat is healthy" vs. "Meat will make you sick"
- "Veganism is healthy" vs. "Veganism will make you sick"
- "Carbs keep you lean" vs. "Carbs make you fat"
- ...and on and on it goes.

Of course, each of the above arguments can be fairly intricate all by itself, regardless which side you're arguing. It's easy to get lost, trying keep up with all of it.

Not to worry, though, because irregardless of all the complex arguments, **I don't think there is a more sound strategy for eating for health (*and* leanness) than the seven words you see above.**

In this chapter I want to break these seven words down, to see just how much there is to the phrase. I'll also talk about one or two slight exceptions worth keeping in mind.

If you're looking for a "solution" or "path" towards a healthy metabolism, it would be encapsulated by those simple seven words:

"Eat food, not too much, mostly plants."

All the information about calories and macros and all the rest... most if it is much ado about nothing. Unless you are getting on a physique stage in the near future, then it's just useless number-crunching that takes you away from the things you *should* be concentrating on.

It takes no time at all to understand, but it will give you a *massive* payoff, and huge rewards, in terms of health, metabolism, and leanness.

In other words, don't let the simplicity fool you.

There is genius in simplicity.

Forget the calorie equations and formulas out there. Contrary to industry gurus, the truth is the human body does not recognize all calories as being equal. In other areas you can say weight is equal: a pound of feathers is equal to a pound of iron because both weigh a pound. But in terms of how your body recognizes and deals with food substances once they enter your body, the equation is not true: 200 calories of a Snickers bar is not recognized, processed, and assimilated in your body the same way 200 calories of asparagus would be.

So let's break down each component part of the brilliant phrase, "Eat food, not too much, mostly plants."

1) Eat Food...

High-quality whole foods serve and always *have* served to balance hormones that regulate your metabolism and gut function. These healthy whole foods also affect the hormones in the brain that are key to controlling appetite and hunger.

This doesn't need to be complicated stuff. You can get into all sorts of details *about* those hormones and neurotransmitters in the brain, but at the end of the day it doesn't much matter. If you eat real, proper food, *that stuff is taken care of.*

Conveniently, it's also easy to tell what is a healthy, whole food, once you throw out any fears you might have from low-carb gurus or whatever. If our ancestors didn't hunt it, gather it, or farm it, then it is not a healthy whole food. Eating a healthy whole food means eating foods in their natural state as much as possible, and with minimal processing.

If it naturally comes from a plant, eat it; if it was "made" *in* a plant, don't. Very seldom is the food (if you can call it that) that you get handed to you from the drive thru ever going to be a healthy whole food.

Ask yourself: How is that food found in nature?

Oh, and also: I hate to disappoint you health nuts here but things like "Almond Milk" are not natural whole foods eaten as found in nature. I've never known of an almond nursing its young with milk. Almonds don't naturally produce milk. Things like "almond milk" are not healthy whole foods as found in nature. It takes processing to get it.

The same is even more true of protein bars and powders and all the rest. Putting the word "engineered" in front of food is a complete marketing stunt. The actual word is "processed." Protein powders and bars are not foods that our ancestors hunted, gathered, or farmed. There isn't a food or meal replacement "product" in the market today that will have the same physiological, hormonally and metabolically balancing effects as actual, natural whole foods. (In fact, they're "engineered" to be hyper-palatable and to fire off reward centers in the brain, to increase your drive to eat more, more, and more. This is what you *don't* want.)

The more ingredients in a food label, then the more that food has been processed, changed and altered. You've probably heard some of this before. Real food seldom even requires a label.

This is often referred to as "the silence of the yams." You don't need to advertise for the potato, and no one does because it's not addictive like hyper-palatable, more marketable foods are, but it is a wonderfully healthy, whole food. In fact, I dedicate a whole chapter of this book to it.

When you see word combinations that begin with "partially" or "un" and then more multi-syllabic, hard-to-pronounce words following that, you know you are not looking at a healthy whole food. The more a food with multiple ingredients tells you how healthy it is… the more suspicious you should be. ("The label doth protest too much.")

Kids breakfast cereals are the obvious example of this. Most people know that a sugary cereal isn't "really" that healthy. The more subtle examples are, as I mentioned above, "health foods" like protein bars, Clif bars, and that kind of thing. They're still engineered and processed, and they won't support long term metabolic health the way real foods will. But they're still marketed to the demographic that is all about "whole foods" and "organic" and the like. But that's all it is: marketing.

You can see this just by checking the labels of so-called "healthy" foods. Almost always, the real healthy whole foods, fresh or frozen, when they do have labels, will have 4-5 ingredients at most.

Finally, I want to add a note about "real" or "natural" foods: don't go too far with this, or take it out of context. This means that **cooking your foods is not only A-OK, it's healthier than eating "raw."** Eating foods "raw" is what's unnatural. I wrote a whole blog post about it, which you can find at scottabelfitness.com/cooking-food-natural/

2) Not Too Much…

After understanding and accepting what "food" is, the next three words of Michael Pollan's excellent axiom of healthy diet-strategy is to eat "not too much."

Does this mean depriving yourself and going hungry? **No!** Not at all. I've been arguing throughout this book *against* extreme deprivation.

What Michael Pollan is referring to here is the something our ancestors couldn't fathom: eating until you are "full" or "stuffed."

In *Beyond Metabolism* I talk a lot about the terms **"justifiable hunger"** and **"tolerable hunger."**

Here's the truth: the natural state of all mammalian creatures on the planet is a state of "tolerable hunger." Watch animals in the wild and they are always foraging for food or hunting prey. Then they rest. It is hard-wired into our brains to look for food, but also hard-wired into our brains that a little bit of hunger equals a whole lot of healthy.

There are hormonal and fancy biological reasons for why this is, but the simple fact of the matter is that a little bit of tolerable hunger keeps you awake, alert, and at your best.

It was not until the advent of extremely convenient hyper-palatable foods (sugar, fat, salt) that man ate until he was full and stuffed. It is not natural or optimal to do so. There is a difference between tolerable hunger (a natural state) and being stuffed (an unnatural state).

Being "stuffed" triggers certain hormones in the brain and gut, creating metabolic and hormonal dysfunction and obstruction.

Unfortunately that "feeling" of being stuffed (especially when it comes from that combo of sugar, salt and fat) acts like a drug, and becomes a habit very quickly.

No one ever overeats on healthy natural whole foods, or gets addicted to them. I constantly hear from clients, "Once I start eating one cookie [or one chip, or one piece of chocolate, or whatever] I just can't stop eating until the whole bag is gone!"

I've never ever heard that said about a bag of apples or skinless chicken breasts.

That, of course, is the other nice thing about Pollan's full axiom I want to mention: if you follow the first part ("eat *food*") and you're eating healthy whole foods, then 90% of the time this second part of the axiom becomes a non-issue. It just takes care of itself. If you eat healthy whole foods, you tend not to eat until you are stuffed, and you learn to accept being a bit hungry while yet having lots and lots of energy.

Genius in simplicity!

So, eat food, but not a lot.

On to the last part…

3) …Mostly Plants

Let me say this again: your exact macro breakdown simply doesn't matter.

I remember when training competitors who were locked into calorie-control nonsense they would break rice cakes or asparagus spears in half in order to "be precise" with calories-control. Talk about breeding potential obsession!

The truth is that if most of your meals are composed of healthy whole foods coming from plants, you will be healthy and lean, without having to obsess about calories and macros and all the rest of it.

Five small meals per day to ensure you are following the rule above of eating food but "not a lot" makes great sense for hormonal balance. Once again modern approaches like IF (Intermittent Fasting) don't properly account for the brain chemistry involved in how hunger is managed and controlled and generated, from the brain to the gut and back again. Sure these concepts are fancy "scientific" stuff (taken out of context), but they fly in the face of optimal hormonal and metabolic reality.

For this part of Pollan's axiom, I'll try to make it a bit simpler: at first, just stick to the "2/3 rule."

Make 1/3 of your plate a protein serving, or a protein and fat serving (like raw nuts), and then make the other 2/3 thirds of your plate plant-based food.

For instance my second meal of the day right now is 40 grams of raw nuts and as much whole fruit as I want, because I'll get satisfied, way before I could get fat. Calories for this meal are *not* an issue. Macro proportions are *not* an issue. My body is smarter than I am in that regard, and so is yours!

Once again, this is not complicated stuff here, and if you need to start somewhere, start with abiding in the mantra "eat food, not too much, mostly plants" and ask yourself, "Is this food choice something my ancestors, hunted, gathered, raised for food or farmed? This leaves your "Clif Bars" and your "Organic Rice and Hemp Seed Protein Powder" out of the equation, and hopefully out of your grocery cart.

Also not that "plant based food" doesn't just mean endless amounts of leafy greens. It means potatoes, rice, legumes, starches — those are all A-OK as well.

Some Exceptions

Now, of course there are exceptions to all simple rules. For instance, not all "man-made" foods are taboo, especially the ones with minimal processing.

One that comes to mind here is **rice cakes** or **corn cakes**.

These foods actually have pretty minimal processing, and can be great choices, especially if limited to only once per day. Some nutritional and fitness gurus will go on and on about the "glycemic index" of rice cakes, and call it a no-no food. But these gurus tend to be the same characters who forbid "carrots" for the same kind of kindergarten-level logic. Rice cakes are very easy to digest and for someone with digestion issues like bloating and stomach distension and the rest, rice cakes once per day can be an especially great choice, as they're very easy on the stomach. Try them, and see how your stomach and your hunger thank you.

Artificial sweeteners are another big example. I choose man-made artificial sweetener over any other "real added sugars" out there, because of the hormonal and metabolic costs of eating such sugars. Sugar comes in many forms and "natural honey" or "raw honey" is still a sugar. Yes "sugar" comes from the sugar cane plant, but in this case it still has to go to the factory for processing before it becomes "sugar," the kind of sugar that can wreak havoc on your hormonal and metabolic balance and function.

Also, before you get all high and mighty about your

artificial sweetener alternative of Stevia, let me remind you that Stevia goes through the exact same processing, starting as a plant and then being processed in a factory. Just because it comes from a plant before being processed into its final form does not make it "superior" except in that it can be marketed that way. It's a way of selling "health consciousness" as an identity. **More on this in the chapter on artificial sweeteners**.

Finally, with my Cycle Diet I do have cheat meals and cheat days where I eat outside my standard diet. I do this for enjoyment. These foods are not exceptions like rice cakes are: I really am eating highly processed foods sometimes. But that's because I do have a sweet tooth, and I enjoy them, and I've structured my diet and timed my refeeds such that within the context of my *overall* diet strategy, they serve their purpose and my personal health and fitness.

* * *

So there, you have it. A diet-strategy to promote health, control weight and get and stay lean as well:

"Eat food, not too much, mostly plants."

And once you factor in what real "food" is, then you know that eating "not too much" doesn't mean deprivation and starvation. Also, you should be aware that as with any rule there is the odd exception here and there (e.g. rice cakes).

I know it's simple, but with those seven words you are well-armed for a starting point in your weight-loss and weight-control goals. None of this is complicated and none of this needs to be. Over-complication offers only the *illusion* of control, but it is mostly wasted effort if you're not four weeks out from a bodybuilding stage. Remember always that "the truth is simple, and simplicity is the truth."

Chapter References

Pollan, Michael. *In Defense of Food: An Eater's Manifesto.* New York: Penguin Press, 2006. Print.

Pollan, Michael. *Food Rules: An Eater's Manual.* New York: Penguin Press, 2009. Print.

Chapter 12.
Routine and Structure

I wanted to include a chapter on routine and structure because although technically it won't help "directly" with your metabolism, it will definitely helping a variety of indirect ways, partly by making things just plain "easier," and also by helping you avoid some of the pitfalls discussed so far (e.g. obsession with calorie counting, focusing too much on what you "can't have," and so on — all of these things will for sure affect things like stress hormones, which will in turn affect metabolism).

It will also help you think and work longterm. As I have repeated ad nauseam throughout this book, any diet *must* be sustainable longterm. If a "diet" is something you do for only 12 weeks, and something that because of its restrictions can really *only* ever be done for some temporary period of time, it will backfire and cause metabolic rebound effects.

Well, a solid routine and structure will help you adopt a diet strategy that *will* work over the long term, and help you "coax" your body to your desired weight loss or weight control goals.

Now, an important note: the point of routine and structure is *not* to create rigid rules and what I call a "diet prison." Just the opposite. The point of routine, structure, regimentation, and ritual is that when a solid diet strategy becomes *habit*, it means you *don't* have to think about it. You don't *need* resistance to "not eat that cookie." Instead, "not eating the cookie" is just a ingrained habit, so that you don't think about it!

Once you control your eating rituals and eating behaviors, that's when you can successfully control your weight long term. Think of them as the foundations of your diet strategy.

Research is showing the faulty mindset of "eat this, not that" is not the key to weight-loss and weight-control. For instance, Professor Rena Wing, a behavioral psychologist at Brown University, and Dr. James Hill, a pediatrician at the University of Colorado founded the National Weight Control Registry to study people who actually had lost weight *and kept it off*.

What'd they find?

Obviously there was some calorie restriction, but there was *no common diet* amongst the thousands of people who'd lost weight and kept it off. The researchers actually noted there was "marked variability" in how successful folks chose to restrict those calories (p. 327). In other words, there was no pattern, no secret, no magic foods to eat and foods to avoid. It wasn't about "eat this, not that." It was about having a sustainable, longterm diet strategy.

What was "really going on" for these successful people was going on beneath the surface. There was a change from "stinkin thinkin" to constructive and empowered thinking, in a way that alters behavior in a sustainable way. The only way to alter behavior in a sustainable way is to not allow it to be subject to self-hate, self-recrimination, self-rejection and the worst of all offenders, self-denial and self-deprivation. Many "eat this, not that" mindsets are steeped in these negative emotions.

These are the kinds of faulty mindsets that lead to faulty behaviours, and faulty behaviours (like attempting "miracle diets" or any metabolically unsustainable diet) are what lead to faulty metabolisms, which in turn lead to yet more of the faulty mindsets in the kind of feedback loop or endless cycle I've been talking about throughout this book.

Sustainable weight-loss is about how you think about food and eating. That is why the North American diet mentality has been such a huge failure, and why the diet industries are built upon the expectation of failure as well. Ask yourself: what's more likely, that you keep going back to Weight-Watchers or Atkins or whatever because "you" keep failing the program, or maybe… there's something inherent in the program that keeps failing you?

I argue the latter. I argue we should reject the whole

notion of this "eat this, not that," mindset.

What the Research Shows About Our Routines

Research shows some other realities that no one wants to admit.

For example, most permanent weight-gain occurs on the weekends. It's not about what they can and cannot stick to during the week, it's about their lifestyle. You could be on Weight Watchers or the HCG diet or even a pretty darn good, reasonable diet, but if you just blow it during the weekends, that'll have consequences.

People will write me and tell me:

- "Well, the weekends are when the kids are off-school and we have to eat out."

- "After a hard week I just want to relax and go out for a nice dinner and have some wine, and what's wrong with that?"

Nothing is wrong with that; this is not a moral issue.

But at the same time — this has nothing to do with the reality of weight-loss. *That is* the challenge: to manage expectations in a realistic way. Eating more than you need to has (cosmetic) consequences. That's not some moral position I'm taking, that's just reality.

Secondary to the above point that most weight is

gained on weekends, researchers found that next in line is that most weight gain occurs during the holiday seasons – notably for Americans, it's during the six weeks from U.S Thanksgiving to New Years.

Weekends and holiday seasons actually combine to account for most weight-gain throughout the year. It's not your carbs, not your macros, not your calories, not your gluten. It's lifestyle. It's habits. It's routine and structure… it is now "routine" for many of us to blow the diet on the weekend (partly because the diet itself is faulty).

The Capital-S Directive

Personally, I follow my Cycle Diet, and I've done so successfully for decades. This means I have one day and *only* day of unstructured eating per week. For me, that day is Sunday.

I've also assigned the following advice to my clients with weight-loss goals: **adopt the "Capital-S" directive.**

This means:

- No **S**nacks
- No **S**econds
- No **S**pirits
- No **S**weets
- No **S**ugars

- No **S**upersizing

- **…except for one day of the week that starts with S**, and only *one* of those days!

(Yes, of course "Special Occasions" as well, but every Friday night, Saturday night and Saturday afternoon don't all count as "Special Occasions.")

That is a successful weight-loss formula. Notice how simple it is, and how when you break it down, a lot of it seems "common sense." (Combine it with Michael Pollan's advice, and you've got a very, very sound diet strategy that isn't too complicated.)

If you have a weight-issue that you want to solve, you may not like the formula above, and you may call it "too restrictive" but it is effective, and realistic. It's about "managing expectations" and "getting real about getting real."

The truth is the average 10 year old now knows all he or she needs to know about healthy eating and weight-control. It's simple, not complicated.

"The truth is simple, and simplicity is the truth!" The truth is that diet-psychology is more important than all the tiny details of nutritional knowledge.

Very few people fail to lose weight or maintain weight-loss because of a lack of knowing "what to eat." People fail because knowing what to do doesn't ensure you'll do it, and they don't do it consistently enough. Everything I've written in this book, any individual tip or suggest or warning—none of it matters if there is no change in behaviour, or no kind of consistency in behaviour.

A healthy metabolism is not about "micromanaging" food macros or gaining more and more nutritional knowledge, or starting some weird metabolism-boosting diet.

Most challenges worth embarking upon are simple in principle, but difficult in practice.

Simple does not mean "easy." But it never means complicated.

It's more comfortable for those who haven't had a breakthrough in weight-loss to believe that the "magic secret" is some specific combination of foods, or some formula that hasn't been discovered yet, or that the secret lies in macronutrient management. That's not the case. The secret is consistency.

The solution is not about this or that food, or this or that diet formulation.

Next you may have to accept that for you, as an individual, your weight-control obstacles are just higher and more frequent. You might have a slower metabolism than that average person. That is definitely true if you're over 40. Or you might just have metabolic damage from ill-advised dieting. But as long as you can accept any of that, or even the possibility of it, *you can still have your own weight-loss breakthrough.*

The metabolic reality is that for some people losing weight will be more difficult than it is for others. That doesn't mean it's impossible. It just means you have to be intelligent and avoid major pitfalls.

I've seen this again and again with my own coaching clients. Plenty of people with genetic or lifestyle obstacles overcome them and achieve their goals. It happens all the time. Every day, in fact.

The reason many people never get there is simply because they don't start with realistic expectations, and I don't just mean expectations about what's possible, but about what the journey will mean in terms of mindset, empowered thinking, psychology and consistency. I mean not embracing what you know, deep down, is the true reality: a magic diet won't do the work for you, but the work can be done.

Manage expectations, learn to embrace structure and follow a few simple rules, make them habits and part of your lifestyle, and you'll find that other things just... fall into place.

Chapter References

De Castro, John M. "Weekly Rhythms of Spontaneous Nutrient Intake and Meal Pattern of Humans." *Physiology & Behavior* (1991): 729–738. Print.

Wing, Rena R, and James O Hill. "Successful Weight Loss Maintenance." *Annual Review of Nutrition* 21 (2001): 323–341.

PART 2
Diet Trends And Diet Truths

Chapter 13.
Metabolic Typing

Lately, as people scramble for attention in the digital world, old fad diets that have long since been debunked are making a new appearance under a different name. But horse manure is still horse manure.

Recently a colleague of mine asked me about "The DNA Diet," a diet I had never heard of. A quick review of the DNA Diet had me almost laughing. People promoting this nonsense couldn't even get their scientific terms correct: one website promoting this nonsense had a heading that read "Insulin Excretion" when they meant to say "Insulin Secretion."

The DNA Diet, is nothing more than a new dressed-up version of "metabolic typing" and its cousin "Eat right for your (blood) type" diet.

The latter was a diet that made the rounds in the late 90s, then was debunked for the nonsense that it is. Well, the DNA Diet is really just a new form of this rubbish.

There will always be the nonsense of diet-cult sleuths who want to exaggerate the "individuality" of human nutritional needs and metabolism — all this "metabolic typing" and so on. In reality, **metabolic individuality is more about nuance and subtlety.** Ethnic and cultural backgrounds can play a role as well.

But these differences certainly *don't* amount to proposing that there are whole subsets of our species that have different macro nutritional requirements than other members of our same species. That's crazy.

Individual metabolic variances exist, absolutely, but they are marginal at best. **Core human macro nutritional requirements are universal. YOU are not a special "case."** Listen to anyone who buys into such nonsense, and they almost always speak like a victim of diet and nutritional circumstance.

When it comes to blood-type diets, this new DNA Diet is fashioned after the academic scientific position on blood type-based diets. Such diets were rather bluntly summarized by Victor Herbert, a hematologist at Mount Sinai Medical Center. When asked in a CNN Interview about diets to suit blood types, his simple response was:

> "The idea is pure horse manure — no relation to reality. The genes for blood type have nothing to do with the genes dealing with the food we eat."

Amen, Victor.

I will use the term "horse manure" for this article…

because it is far more polite than the words I would normally choose to describe the nonsense of the DNA Diet.

As I mentioned, like most diet-fads that try to pretend to be "scientific" (hear that Paleo?) the blood-type diet had its moment in the sun in the late 1990s, then faded into obscurity as most diet fads are wont to do. But every so often it makes a blip again on the radar of pop-culture. The DNA Diet is one such blip: same lame argument, same lame logic.

Real science does lend some weight to arguments about what we know about food, diets, and gene expression. For instance, in the past 15 years, geneticists have identified a very long list of "genes" that affect the metabolism of carbs, fats, and proteins. The majority of these genes exist in *all* humans, even other primates, for that matter. What this means is that macronutrient needs of all humans are basically the same!

Epidemiological research is pretty clear about this.

As I said, genetically based individual differences in the metabolism of proteins, carbs, and fats do exist, but they are *subtle*. None of the real research on blood genes, or genes to do with food and eating… none of that research supports metabolic typing diets, eat right for your blood type diets, or the latest in pseudo-science nonsense, the "DNA" Diet.

All of these fad diets feed the misinformed fury of the so-called "importance of macronutrient profiling" which is just more diet and fitness industry nonsense, and more of the "the illusion of control" I've talked about.

The real truth is that a diet-strategy that follows healthy guidelines toward whole unprocessed foods, composed mostly of plants, including grains and starches like potatoes, rice, and so on, is all anyone really needs to eat right for "your type."

Chapter 14.
Realistic Protein Needs

What is the right amount of protein for someone looking to lose weight (or add muscle, or what-have-you)?

What's optimal for metabolic function?

Marketers would have you believe that to build a physique you require "more protein."

They would also have you believe that it's unlikely you can get this high quality protein that you need from diet alone. They just happen to have "engineered food protein" in a powder that is of the highest quality, better than food, actually — you really need it. Or they like to "insinuate" that if you are truly "serious" about your commitment to physique enhancement then you need protein powder – and you need their protein powder.

Wait a minute.

Engineered food is really just another name for processed food made in a factory. Real research on protein has something *different* to say about your protein needs. The problem of course is that a lot of popular "knowledge" on our protein requirements comes from completely biased sources.

Protein Marketing Tactics

When I served on the board of advisers for several supplement companies (companies whose millions of dollars were primarily made with two products – protein powders and fat burners) there were several marketing tactics that were always used because they always worked.

One of these lame tactics was to write articles "rating the protein powders."

Maybe you recall seeing these articles in various magazines. Maybe you've seen such article on various websites. They still exist today.

The point of these "rate the protein powders" went beyond just trying to get you to see Brand X as the "best" brand. That is the simple and easy scam to recognize. (I wrote some of them.)

Below the surface of these "rate the protein powders" articles there is a broader agenda. You have to remember where these articles are placed: in industry magazines and on industry websites where the consumer wants to be an informed member of the sub-culture.

The unconscious message delivered in these "rate the

protein powder" articles is as follows:

4) Protein powders are very important parts of your eating and training regimen.

5) You need to be taking protein powder.

6) If you really care about "results" then you need to take the "*right*" protein powder.

By writing articles like "rate the protein powders" you REMOVE the question in the consumer's minds of whether protein powders are even necessary to begin with. You see the intention in all of this. With the question of "Do I really need this?" removed from your mind, then the answer becomes "of course I need this" and then you are likely now a buyer of Brand X protein powder.

So, let's ask the question then:

If you are serious about building and sculpting your physique, do you "really" need "extra" protein at all, let alone in the form of processed powder made in a factory?

Actual Research On Your Protein Needs

What does the research say about protein needs for muscle growth and optimal metabolic function?

Quite simply, the latest research has debunked the notion of that you need more protein to build muscles, or that you need it at certain times, or whatever other doggerel is being sold.

Yes, if you're resistance training, there certainly *is* an advantage to eating 'a bit more' than the recommended daily intake 0.8 grams of protein per kilo of bodyweight, but you don't need much more than that.

Studies at McMaster University provided diets to participants of either 1.35 or 2.62 grams of protein per kilogram of bodyweight. The participants were untrained men who were subjected to one month of intensive weight-training at 90 minutes daily, six days per week.

Both groups gained muscle size and strength, as you'd expect, but those who consumed the larger amount of protein gained no more than those participants who took in barely half as much. Moreover, the gains of these subjects should be attributed to physiological adaptation to training stimulus. Having been previously untrained, and then going from zero to 90 minutes daily 6 days per week would certainly cause a physiological adaptation response, and the result would of course be noticeable muscle growth and strength. The fact is that with training, it is well-established that most trainees will make their most significant gains within the first six months to a year of training (provided that the training protocol is adequate and the intensity of workout effort is moderate or greater).

Furthermore, the research also shows that experienced bodybuilders who have already developed their physiques actually need *less* protein to maintain that muscle mass. Read that again. Experienced bodybuilders need *less* protein to maintain.

At the height of my career I was 260 lbs, and under 10% bodyfat. I consumed about half as much protein as the pros I knew around me, and I never took a protein powder supplement. My muscles didn't waste away.

But why would bodybuilders with established physiques need "less" protein? That seems counter-intuitive doesn't it? They need less protein because of the amazing wisdom of the body. They need less protein because over time, this form of resistance training teaches the body to retain more protein from the diet. Kind of like prioritizing what kind of fuel it needs. Our bodies adapt, and this is no exception.

The dirty little secret that the supplement industry doesn't want you to know is that massive protein intake would work *against* this physiologically constructive adaptation response!

Excessive protein intake increases protein turnover rates and this creates a kind of dependency on continual excessive protein intake. This means that in a well-developed bodybuilder physique, the more protein taken in, the more protein is *wasted*, and thus the more is in turn needed from diet (creating yet another feedback loop).

More isn't always better: yes, agreed, a little more protein is good for the hard training resistance trainee. A lot more is nonsensical and unnecessary.

As I have argued in many, many previous articles, it's the protein sparing macronutrients (fats and carbs) that require the most attention in any diet. My coaching clients know this. You can either focus on one or the other of these protein sparing macronutrients, or hey, even both! It doesn't matter.

When you do, calories from fats and/or carbs should be at least two to three times higher than protein calories. This is why I mentioned the "2/3s" rule in Chapter 11:

> Make 1/3 of your plate a protein serving, or a protein and fat serving (like raw nuts), and then make the other 2/3 thirds of your plate plant-based food.

This "spares" protein to be used to build and rebuild tissue, and it teaches the body to use protein more efficiently as well. My description of the two-thirds rule probably favours carbs, slightly, but the fats are still there.

Chapter 15.
Paleo I

First of all, make no mistake that **the Paleo Diet is founded on the heels of Atkins.**

That is pretty clear if you read the material available regarding both approaches to food and eating. This means it maintains some of the original biases and mistakes of Atkins as well. And, more to the point, both these diets seem to induce a type of religious fervor once they enter into the pop-culture consumer consciousness.

This makes them especially dangerous, since what people want to believe to be true has more power than what is actually true… at least in the cultural zeitgeist.

And to be honest and open here, the dogma of fad diets as religions is simply a turn-off to real researchers seeking truth.

It gets tiring being bombarded with and asked about

fad diet religion nonsense, over and over again:

> Low-fat, low-carb, high-protein, vegan, macros, high-protein, Zone, Atkins, Paleo, Mediterranean, gluten-free, low-glycemic, raw food, no starch, alkaline, detoxes and cleanses, Metabolic Typing, DNA Diets, Isagenics, Body by V

...and all the rest of are religious 'denominations' of diet religion fantasy.

What applies across the board when it comes to fad diet religions is that people believe what they want to believe. For proof, just say something critical in social media about whatever current vogue diet-culture trend is gaining traction and watch their attack dog followers come out in droves.

I've experienced this many times.

My point is that it illustrates how much this is more about emotional identity membership than about any kind of science of nutrition.

And Paleo is no different.

People have a 'need to be right' when it comes to their own version of what healthy eating is.

And make no mistake, modern fad diet religions love to use the claim of "science and research" as their bible. The only problem with this is that so often their science and research is sketchy at best. It's often taken completely out of context (as Atkins does regarding the glycemic index) or flat out wrong. And in the case of the poor poor Peter Paleo Pundit, the science is just plain wrong, as I have pointed out in my previous articles. Moreover, it is so often the case that the founders of these fad diet religions are themselves not qualified in the area of "proof" that they offer for their diet agenda – as we will see below in the case of Paleo diet religion and its creator God, Loren Cordain.

Debunking the Paleo Diet from the Outside-In

Ah yes, so here is faithful the Peter Paleo Pundit or dieter, an 'expert' in nutrition who follows the Paleo bible. He goes out with his family for brunch and orders scrambled eggs with bacon and spinach. No cheese allowed with that because according to the Paleo bible, humans have only been eating cheese for 8,000 years, and of course this is much too recent on the evolutionary scale to be good for us, don't you know.

And while that brunch meal is normally served with home fried potatoes, well, Peter Paleo doesn't eat those either, since humans have only been eating potatoes for 14,000 years, and yet again, this is far too recent to be healthy according to the Paleo bible doctrine.

A side of toast would certainly go nice with eggs, but Peter, as a good Paleo evangelist tries to educate and Paleo Preach to everyone at his table by pointing out that he won't eat the bread either because we all should know how bad wheat is for us and it's only been part of human diets for 10,000 years or so. This also according to Paleo Diet bible chapters is way too recent to be good for us.

So Peter Paleo Preacher adheres to the "lessons" taught and preached in his Paleo Bible.

The only problem with Peter's logic is that it's simply not true.

The God of Paleo

The person known as the creator of Paleo is Loren Cordain, someone with no formal training as a paleobiologist or evolutionary biologist.

This is the kind of expertise that often flows out of the fitness, diet, and supplement industries. Think of Suzanne Somers, for instance, as "a supplement expert."

The thing is, real experts from these fields of study (experts in how Paleolithic humans actually ate, and lived) have now stepped forward and discredited many of the core ideas and central tenets of the "Paleo bible."

Such sacrilege! Say it ain't so! It's nutritional religious blasphemy I tell you – heresy to go against the bible of Paleo!

But, in her **2013 TED Talk** for instance, biomolecular archeologist Christina Warinner of the University of Zurich said, "This version of the Paleo diet that's promoted in popular books, on TV, on self-help websites, and in the overwhelming majority of press has no basis in archeological reality."

Then she dismantled Paleo diet religious nonsense point by point.

Watch it here: **http://youtu.be/BMOjVYgYaG8**

Let's look at some of the facts that explode the biblical commandments of Paleo God and creator Loren Cordain:

- There is plenty of evidence that even before the agricultural revolution, humans ate seeds and grains, and there is new evidence that Neanderthals and Paleolithic humans ate barley, beans, and a variety of tubers. In short, as always, humans ate what was available to them, and **humans learned to process and refine foods well before the agricultural age** (the era so central to the Paleo argument, other than the Paleolithic era itself of course).

- Furthermore, proceedings of the National Academy of Sciences published a set of four research papers that demonstrated human ancestors known as hominids, living 2-3 MILLION years ago ate, more grasses **AND GRAINS** than they did fruits and leaves.

- Moreover, as many experts in the field of study of ancient humans have also pointed out, pretty much every single food that Paleolithic humans consumed are foods that no longer even exist today. Every food we eat today in our modern world is different than the foods eaten by

Paleolithic ancestors.

In fact a look at what our ancestors ate makes it fairly obvious that modern humans couldn't eat the same way our ancestors ate 20,000 years ago, even if we wanted to.

But then... there is the psychological considerations of... why would we want to?

If Paleolithic humans had a choice, they wouldn't have wanted to eat that way, either!

No one ever seems to consider such a question relevant. But of course it is relevant. Because there is the matter of completely neglecting the reality of whether our ancestors enjoyed their survival diets or found them pleasurable. There is ample evidence that they did not. In fact, **experts suggest Paleolithic humans HATED their survival diets**, which is precisely why they began experimenting with their foods to begin with: processing and refining their food to make it more pleasurable and palatable. **That is also an innate characteristic of being human**. To suggest humans ate this way because it was "natural" for them and therefore "better" is just a huge leap of logic that makes no sense.

The very moment humans learned to make tools, and to refine and process and cook their food... THEY DID SO. IMMEDIATELY.

Seems "diet-psychology" was also present that far back. So once again we witness the limitations and outright "errors" of pop-cultural diet fads represented as "scientific." And, even worse, they're taking on ridiculous religious cult-like followings. So once again we see the sleight of hand magician's trick of duping consumers.

Because in the final analysis by real and qualified experts, **the Paleo Diet is not at all what it claims to be,** nor can it do what it claims to do, nor are its scientific arguments (it's bible) even accurate.

(Pssst… hear that Crossfitters!)

As Fitzgerald said in his book:

> "Crossfitters who embrace the Paleo Diet, and Paleo Dieters who embrace Crossfit, like to believe that 'reason and intelligence' lead them to these associations. But in fact, the pipeline between these two cults has nothing to do with truth."

The Paleo Diet merely builds on Atkins and borrows a lot of the same faulty arguments as well. But to claim that the era of agriculture is what led to modern obesity and weight-issues is just… plain… WRONG.

But poor, poor pitiful Peter, the Paleo Pundit continues to preach and live by a diet religion based on a faulty research premise.

In short, he thinks his diet is science-based, when it is faith-based.

Chapter 16.
Paleo II

Part 1 explored the Paleo Diet Religion from the outside-in.

Paleolithic humans were not lean because of what they ate (another point often insinuated in the Paleo Religious dogma). Humans were lean because of how they lived, and because of the harsh conditions of being human in earlier epochs of human history.

You would think that would be obvious, when you compare their lives to our modern ones of abundance, and the modern provisions of heat, food and shelter we enjoy.

But this is how diet fad religions work. They twist common sense to the point of laughable absurdity, all the while trying to make an argument that is supposedly based in science and research. But as I illustrated in Part

1, the science and research supporting "The Paleo Diet" is just plain in error, so you are left to take The Paleo Diet on faith, as any hapless religious follower should do.

It's an aspect of sub-culture more generally: when it comes to "diets," **any diet fad is a fad when it becomes "a movement."**

But like most "movements" these fad diet religions go only so far and then stop, hence the literal meaning of the term "a movement." They stop because they are simply wrong, and they don't work.

Remember that what "works" must be defined in the long-term: diets must not just be "doable" but also sustainable in a pleasurable way as well.

Members of the fad diet-religions believe they are eating more sensibly than you or I, and that their diet god is the one and only "true" diet god. But just like religions of spirituality, fad diet religious followers are just eating more ritualistically.

There is "ritual" in what they do, and that is one of its main draws among consumers who don't know any better.

In this case, poor misinformed Paleo dieters see not eating starches as necessary to health and well-being, when actually this is just a sacrament of the Paleo diet.

It is just like those who want to develop their bodies, and think that their special brand of protein shake (taken at such and such a time) is a vital key to their development, yet really it's just a sacrament to being a consumer in that particular sub-culture.

In today's culture, a person's identity formation has more to do with fad diet popularity than anyone wants to admit. Consumers want to think that their diet-adherence is based in research and science, when it's likely based in faith and other ritualistic behaviors that go with it.

Here, let's Debunk Paleo from the Inside-Out:

The Actual Food and Eating Claims of the Paleo Diet

One of the prominent "food" claims made by Paleo purists is that a diet of 50% red meat is healthier than a diet with less meat. But in 2012, the Harvard School of Public Health released a study that shows that the more red meat people eat... the sooner they die.

Also popular with Paleo pundits and other modern pop-diet experts is the claim that a diet without dairy is healthier than a diet that includes dairy. But 2010 research from Cardiff University in Wales showed that eating more dairy products was associated with lower risk of heart disease, stroke, diabetes, and death by any cause.

In the Paleo religious "bible" the argument is that a diet that excludes all grains is healthier than one that includes whole grains. (Bashing grains is the "sodium demon" of our generation, and of Paleo in particular. Grains are the Satan of the Paleo bible.) And yet The National Institute of Health's AARP Diet and Health

Study, a MASSIVE research undertaking that tracked the death and disease rates of half a million men and women over 9 years, found that those who ate THE MOST whole grains were 22% LESS LIKELY to die during this 9 years period than those who ate less whole grains. Furthermore, the people with THE MOST consumption of whole grains were about 30% LESS LIKELY to develop heart disease.

So much for the Paleo diet and avoiding grains being "healthier."

Clearly, the research just does not bear out the claims made by Paleo. So once again, as any good religious follower, *you have to go on faith.*

But here's the thing, as with most "diet religions," of course Paleo Preaching Pundits will turn critics into skeptics, into "non-believers" and "outsiders" if you will.

And when research doesn't support a fad diet religion-du-jour? Why, then what you do is attack the researchers!

This tactic is alive and well in the modern fitness and diet industries.

I've been on the receiving end of attacks from zealots many times in my career.

Any research that doesn't support a fad diet religion like Paleo "must be" tainted by food industry interests. It's a conspiracy!

And yet as I showed in Part 1, the Paleo God, and Paleo's creator, has no background at all as a paleobiologist or evolutionary biologist. His arguments are just flat out incorrect!

This whole fitness and diet industry conspiracy theory nonsense is getting really, really old and stale. What we witness here in the religion of Paleo is the long-standing cultural tradition of all vogue diet cults and trends that I've lived long enough to keep witnessing again, and again, and again.

Let's be honest:

If there is a "paradigm blindness" at work here… it is probably NOT with academic research, but more likely with the evangelists who continue to promote, prop up, and push an agenda based in opinion – even when the research is to the contrary on a point by point basis – as it is in the fad diet Paleo arguments.

But instead of dealing with the research, it is much easier for these diet zealots to simply attack the credibility of the researchers and yell "conspiracy."

Really?

Let's tear down the idea that grains are "evil" some more.

Professor Ann Stone of Arizona State University has demonstrated that humans from populations with high-starch diets typically have more copies of the gene that regulates the production of the enzyme amylase, an enzyme that aids starch digestion.

What this shows is that humans living in areas where

grain agriculture was adapted at the beginning of the Neolithic period evolved pretty darn quickly to **BENEFIT** from a grain-focused diet.

Once again, contrary to Paleo arguments, research like Professor Stone's illustrate that when it comes to diet adaptation, human evolution as an omnivore species is not always slow – a fact that flies in the face of the religious dogma of the Paleo Diet.

Other research also shows that the human species was quick to adapt to increased grain consumption, suggesting that **the human's capacity for genetic adaptations to all kinds of diets, foods and environments is one of the factors that allowed our species to thrive and spread across the globe.**

Eating grain is not "unnatural." It is merely a reflection of the evolution of our omnivore species, and of our ability to adapt.

Modern nutrition "lore" (that is, the kind preached by Paleo religious zealots) has posited that eating grains causes systemic inflammation and other related issues, including "cognitive impairment" often labeled as "grain brain."

But the ACTUAL research (and an abundance of it I may add), shows that people around the world who consume the most whole grains actually have LOWER levels of systemic inflammation. (For instance, Lefevre, M et al, "Effect of whole grains on markers of subclinical inflammation," *Nutrition Review*, July 2012)

What we see here is that there is a cycle of fad diet

religiosity that takes hold of pop-culture every few years. The Paleo diet is just one of the latest examples. Atkins came before it. But these fad diet religions are seldom based in hard science and accredited research. People come to believe in them based on little more than the rudimentary elements of "faith" and "psychology."

Paleo has been debunked over and over again... but the books continue to sell. I even saw "Paleo Diet for Women" the other day at the bookstore, as if to imply that one gender should of course eat differently, and that one gender has different metabolic needs than the other, even though we are both of the same species and evolution. So by that logic your female German Shepherd needs to eat differently than your male German Shepherd, and the male lion must have to eat a different "kill" than the female lion, and so on.

But of course, I am just an outsider skeptic, a non-believer, non-follower, a Paleo "atheist" if you will.

And for that I thankfully say AMEN!

Chapter 17.
The REAL "Low-Carb" Diet

Most of what you've been sold about "low carbs diets" is incomplete.

Personally, I am not a fan of low-carbs diets to begin with... and even that is when they are done right. But what is passing for a "low carbs diet" now doesn't even come close to the original intention or use of the low carb approach. I'm going to discuss the reality of low-carbs diets.

Since I don't use low carb approaches, in the second part of this chapter I'll talk about my friend and colleague Kevin Weiss who at competition time (and *only* at competition time) follows the "true and authentic" low-carbs approach to lose weight, make his weight class, and lift like a champion. (And oh, he's only a World Champion in Raw powerlifting, and hugely successfully champion natural bodybuilder as well.)

Low Carbs: What you NEED to Know

In the last two years I've devoted a fair amount of my research time to a specific niche of nutritional science.

I've been studying the "history" of various diets... how they came to be, how they came to be marketed, and what the real truth of modern nutrition is, based upon what nutritional science history reveals to us.

I've learned that the "low-carbs diets nonsense" so many people have bought into is not what the true intentions of the low-carbs diet approach was originally meant to be.

If you are considering a low carb diet right now, more than likely you want to follow a low carbs diet-approach for cosmetic reasons. For others, you might have been fed so much junk science about carbs that you want to follow a low-carbs diet because you are 'afraid' of carbs. And that too has a lot to do with the history of diet trends.

In the 1970s the "low-fat" diet approach was the vogue trend and all the rage. Like any trend it had its victors. I myself to this day generally follow a low-fat, higher carbs approach (but I want to add that there are no one size fits all diet agendas... minus a few generalizations like Michael Pollan's axiom).

In the 70s, a decade of "low-fat" madness didn't work for everyone, but it did make people "afraid" of fats as a fuel source. (Remember that as we move forward now.)

Before there was Atkins, there was always talk in esoteric medical journals about an alternative approach to dieting – as a way to treat various brain disorders (specifically, epilepsy). This diet-approach to "treatment" was referred to as "the extremely high fat diet approach" for treatment. Look at that phrase carefully. This is where diet-psychology and marketing comes into play. It also is where something becomes "mutated" from one purpose to another, and twisted to fit some marketing agenda, even if it violates the rules and principles this thing is founded upon. And such was the case for the "low-carbs diet" approach, which was originally the "high fat" approach. Yes, there is a difference.

Notice how I put "diet" after the low-carbs phrase: because this is where all the nonsense ensues.

Diet Industry Quandary

In the wake of the low-fat diet revolution, there was a fear associated with the word "fat" as a nutritional component (much like there is fear associated with carbs today).

Those professionals who believed strongly in a possible benefit for the "extremely high fat diet" approach… well, they had a dilemma. There was no way to "convince" the consumer, who had been led to fear "fats," that there was a benefit to "extremely high fat" as an approach to weight-control.

When you want to make money selling a diet "revolution" (as Atkins called it) you can't do it by getting people to buy into a notion of a sudden 180 degree psychological flip from "low-fat" dieting (because fat is evil and makes you fat) and then expect them to believe an "extremely high fat diet" is suddenly the key to weight control.

The Difference Between "Extremely High Fat" and "Low Carbs"

To make a long story short, the Atkins generation skirted around the intent of the "actual" extremely high fat diet approach. "High-fat" was scary, but the term "low carbs" diet made more sense.

Just like "low fat" made fat the enemy to be feared for weight-gain, marketers did the same by coining the term "low carbs." The only problem with this is that the term "low carbs" is actually disingenuous to the REAL purpose of the extremely high fat diet approach.

The original notion of extremely high fat diets, was all about its effects on brain chemistry for people with brain disorders like epilepsy. It was never supposed to be about health, nutrition, weight-loss or metabolism. Those are just diet-industry created notions. Historically, the reason medical experts were emphasizing this diet was because of the influence of extremely high fats on the brain – and not because of the "low carbs" on the other side of that equation. It was also extremely demanding, and really only implemented in medical settings.

The Low Carbs Diet is NOT a

"High Protein" Diet!

You see Atkins and the rest of these diet pushers couldn't sell a diet-agenda that suggests it is "extremely demanding" or that it should be followed in a medical/hospital setting. That is no way to make money in the diet industry. So they just ignored this stuff.

What ended up happening was a misinterpretation of the 'extremely high fat diet' as a new 'low carbs diet.' Since most dieters and pop-culture followers of "nutrition" were still convinced that "fat" was a bad word, instead of praising fat they vilified carbs. Dieters were now fearful of both carbs and fats, and the result is the complete misapplication of the low-carb diet, which was always meant to be an extremely high fat diet.

"Protein-Sparing Nutrients"

You see the whole notion of a low carbs diet is that it can only work and work properly if fats are not only high, but EXTREMELY HIGH.

A low carb diet was never meant to be a high protein diet.

Because people were misled to fear both carbs and fats, the whole low-carbs diet approach ended up becoming a high-protein diet, and protein was sold as some kind of miracle macronutrient.

If you try to follow this faulty version of the low carb diet, where "low carb" = "high protein and medium fats," you'll **usually pay a high metabolic price for**

making this mistake. Don't even get me started on the side-effects of a mis-applied ketogenic or low carbs diets. It's a mess of digestive issues and other metabolic and health consequences. (You can look up "side effects of keto-diets" for yourself... just do so on reputable sites like Pub-Med or something.)

Basic nutritional biochemistry teaches that carbs and fats are meant to be "protein *sparing* nutrients." This means that EITHER or BOTH carbs and fats must be high enough in the diet to allow protein to be "spared" and used to build and rebuild tissue as it is meant to do.

It's this purpose and the nitrogen component of protein that makes protein special to begin with. But a high protein diet usually means that either fats or carbs are not high enough, and this produces more harm than good.

For the actual, original "extremely high fat diet approach" that the low-carb diet is supposed to be, the percentage of fat in the diet needs to be upward of 70% fats. In truth, the "low carbs" approach, when it is done correctly, it is actually a very low protein diet.

Enter Kevin Weiss' Approach

World Powerlifting Champ Kevin Weiss and I get together at least once per week for coffee. At our last get together I could tell Kevin had dropped a couple lbs.

"Back on the high-fat diet?" I asked him.

"Yep," he said.

You see Kevin is just several weeks out from the next World Championships and he wants to make weight for a lighter weight class. And when dieting, Kevin – who is a natural "meat tooth" (in contrast to my "sweet tooth") – he always opts for the extremely high-fat diet approach.

Now with Kevin, I would never ask "So, you back to low carbs diet?"

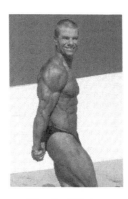

Kevin Weiss

That would be like an insult to him. Kevin is an astute student of the game. He knows that the term "low carb diet" has no relevance to what he is doing: it's the extremely high fat diet that is more descriptive of his approach.

This is the mistake 99% of people out there make. Over coffee, Kevin explained to me why he gave up trying to help people with this diet: "Scott, they just won't take their fats high enough to make it work long-term."

Kevin's Weight-Loss Competition Diet

So how does he do it? Kevin needs to drop some weight but still be able to perform at his best. If you buy into industry nonsense you would think that since Kevin is a powerlifter his emphasis would be on getting in enough protein. WRONG.

His emphasis is in getting in a high enough amount of fat.

In fact only 12% of his calories come from protein! That's right: 12% Protein! Much less than even I advice in my diets (which are usually about 40% protein, 40% carbs, 20% fats).

Read on. This is what the "low carbs diet approach" was supposed to be all along, an extremely, *extremely* high-fat diet.

I got Kevin to scribble down his meals for the day for me, but I'll only show you two. I had a great laugh out loud moment. Check this "weight-loss" diet:

Breakfast:

3 whole eggs

4 slices bacon

4 tablespoons sour cream

2 slices cheddar cheese

2 tablespoons butter

½ cup heavy cream

Lunch

2 cups spinach

1 avocado

3 oz. regular ground beef

4 tablespoons olive oil

1 slice cheddar cheese

Meal Alternative

2 teaspoons coconut oil

4 ounces prime rib

3 whole eggs

1 cup spinach

½ cup feta cheese

½ cup heavy cream

4 tablespoons sour cream

Okay, so you get the picture. The true essence of a low-carbs approach that can actually work and not negatively impact metabolism is that it is *extremely* high in fat. On a lark, we decided to breakdown his macros:

Protein:

less than 13%

Carbs:

5%

Fat:

a whopping 82%.

Then Kevin corrected this by saying he forgot that later that day he was hungry, so he had a whole avocado with cream cheese. This skews his macros even more, meaning his protein was less than 12%, and his fats were even higher than 82%.

THIS, my friends, is what the real low-carb diet looks like. (Doesn't look that much like the one you see on grocery store magazine racks, does it?) Fitness industry twits try to tweak the science of this and turn it into a *moderate* fat, high protein, low carbs diet. This was never the original structure of "the extremely high fat diet approach."

The *consequence* of twisting this diet into a high protein, medium fat, low carbs diet is that it is metabolically destructive and creates a host of digestive issues to boot.

Metabolic Shift

Let's not forget the metabolic shift involved in going to an extremely high fat approach. Kevin is quick to point out that when switching to his greater than 82% fat diet – the calories must be high at first to accomplish the "metabolic shift" involved with processing fats.

Kevin knows what he's doing! He pays no attention to industry vogue trends. He follows the "low carbs diet" as it was *originally* designed and intended. He's already noticeably losing weight, and his digestion is fine, his performance fine his fine, and the degree of difficulty for diet-compliance for him? Negligible.

The reason industry consumers get into so much trouble with trying to go "low carbs" is because it's been twisted; unless you are willing to go extremely, extremely high fat then you should trash any notion of thinking low carbs is right for you.

Remember that even when it's done right, the extremely high fat diet is VERY demanding and extremely difficult to follow. If you look at medical websites, they'll also comment that such a diet would be suited to a *very limited* proportion of the general public. I'd keep that in mind whenever you consider the "low carb approach," and realize that diets like Paleo, Atkins, and South Beach are marketing "mutations" of the original low-carb diet. (Mutations that were made not for any scientific reason, but for the historical and marketing reasons discussed above.)

The low carb approach, when the fats are high

enough, is both difficult and very demanding. When it is just moderate fat and high protein, it's dangerous, and certainly not good for the metabolism long term!

Chapter 18.
Gluten

I've been talking a lot about how studying the history of nutrition yields a lot of useful information and patterns. You start noticing cycles. There is an ebb and flow to basic ideas coming and going, just with new names or buzzwords attached.

In a past chapter we saw that the DNA Diet was just a new version of the "eat right for your blood type" or "metabolic typing" nonsense from way back. We also saw how Paleo is in many ways just an off-shoot of Atkins.

The current fear of gluten is similar. It is the re-emergence of a common idea. That is, over the years there have been many nutritional phantom creations that are made out to be the real "root" causes of any possibly symptom you may happen to have. But that's all they are: phantoms. They don't exist; they're not really there. Most of the time the symptoms can be put down to something much simpler: *stress* (in its various forms), but instead they're attributed to this or that specific food item.

With gluten we've reached new depths of insanity: there are now gluten-free dating sites and gluten-free food for dogs. Gluten-hysteria has more than taken off. But as with the DNA Diet, the gluten boogeyman is something we've seen before.

Some of you may recall when a book called *The Yeast Connection* made some silly leaps in its conclusions. The author used a very general symptomology of malaise, and soon had a whole bandwagon of people self-diagnosing and self-treating a non-existent disease. Instead of "gluten" it was "candida albicans."

In other words... yeast.

Yeast was the nutritional cause of *all* your symptoms, even the mental and emotional ones. Only it turned out this wasn't true in any way, shape, or form. Of course, you couldn't convince the hundreds of thousands of the book's believers of that.

In 2002, German researchers published a comprehensive review of the accumulated research about candida/yeast. Over one hundred relevant, peer-reviewed studies were analyzed. The authors wrote, "Neither epidemiological nor therapeutic studies provide any evidence for the existence of the so-called 'Candida-syndrome' or 'Candida-hypersensitivity-syndrome'" (see Lacour). Since then, the whole matter of yeast/candida and its contribution to ill-health has been so debunked and disproven that it now also appears on the

"Quackwatch" website.

Gluten is simply a new nutritional scapegoat. The form remains the same. Whatever your issue, from constipation to diarrhea to headaches, ADD, infertility, joint pain and depression: going gluten-free is the treatment. It just so happens that these general and broad symptoms are eerily similar to symptoms of "candida-hypersensitivity syndrome" from a decade or two ago.

Surveys have shown that the majority of people who buy gluten-free foods *can't even tell you why they do so*. Late night talk show TV host Jimmy Kimmel did a segment on this. He asked people who maintained a gluten-free diet what gluten was, and the answers were hilarious. The segment illustrated the way North Americans follow nutritional trends with little to no knowledge of the facts.

You may not know the science of what gluten is, but you just sort of know "it's bad for you." This is how nutritional scapegoating works. It's how the whole movement took off a decade or two ago. Yet, as with the "yeast connection," gluten-sensitivity has been debunked.

Biesiekierski et al. (see "No effects") found that only 8% of self-diagnosed gluten-sensitive individuals experienced a worsening of symptoms when gluten was added to their diets. So while Celiac is a very real issue, and a painful one at that, and gluten-sensitivity "can" certainly exist, *the reality of it is that actual gluten-sensitivity itself is extremely rare*.

In 2012 Italian researchers wrote "that 'sense' should prevail over 'sensibility' to prevent a gluten preoccupation from evolving into the conviction that gluten is toxic for most of the population. We must prevent a possible health problem from becoming a social health problem" (See Di Sabatino). What with gluten-free dating websites and

Back in the 50s and most of the 60s the average North American got up to 30% of daily calories from bread. There was a plate of bread on the table for virtually every meal, with the exception of lunch, when sandwiches were often the daily fare anyway. If there was a gluten problem back then it would have been a massive epidemic. But there wasn't, because gluten is not a problem for most of the population.

To my mind, rising stress levels are more the trigger to gastrointestinal issues than any other cause, other than direct food allergies.

We live in an era where you are led to believe any symptoms are a consequence of incorrect nutrition, even when you are already obsessed with eating healthy. But this is just nutritional scapegoating at its height. Much of the time it is the stress *about* eating healthy that is causing the issues in the first place!

To put it bluntly, it is very likely that unless you have full-blown celiac disease, you have no real issue with gluten. It won't upset you, and it won't mess up your metabolism.

Finally, here's an interesting note about the way science works, but which you don't hear about as much. (It does get reported, but disappears in the mainstream.)

The very researchers who suggested "non-celiac gluten sensitivity" in the first place actually did another study. (This is the Biesiekierski et al. "No Effects" study I mentioned above.) One of the team researchers, Peter Gibson, wrote "In contrast to our first study ... we could find absolutely no specific response to gluten" (qtd. in Welsh).

In other words, they checked and attempted to replicate their own work, but were unable to do so. There was *no specific response to gluten*. This is because real scientists like Gibson look both to prove and *dis*prove their results. Note the lack of an agenda here. In fact, just to be sure, the researchers replicated *again* with a third study (see Biesiekierski et al. "Characterization). Again, no negative response to gluten was found!

Long story short: if you don't have Celiac disease, you can enjoy gluten-filled meals. Be wary of self-diagnosing, and if something seems like nutritional scapegoating, it probably is.

Chapter References:

Biesiekierski, Jessica R et al. "No Effects of Gluten in Patients with Self-Reported Non-Celiac GlutenSensitivity After Dietary Reduction of Fermentable, Poorly Absorbed,Short-Chain Carbohydrates." *Gastroenterology* 145.2 (2013): 320–328.e3.

Biesiekierski, J R et al. "Characterization of Adults with a Self-Diagnosis of Nonceliac Gluten Sensitivity."

Nutrition in Clinical Practice 29.4 (2014): 504–509. Web.

Di Sabatino, A. et al, "Nonceliac gluten sensitivity: sense of sensibility?" *Annals of Internal Medicine* (Feb 2012).

Dube, SR. et al, "Cumulative childhood stress and autoimmune disease in adults," *Psychosomatic Medicine* 71.2 (Feb 2009).

Lacour, Michael et al. "The Pathogenetic Significance of Intestinal Candida Colonization -- a Systematic Review From an Interdisciplinary and Environmental Medical Point of View." *International Journal of Hygiene and Environmental Health* (2002): 205–257–268.

Sapone, A et al "Divergence of gut permeability and mucusol immune gene expression in two gluten-associated conditions: celiac disease and gluten sensitivity," *BMC Medical Journal* (March 2011)

Van Dyke, CT, et al "Increasing Incidence of celiac disease in North American Population," *American Journal of Gastroenterology* (May 2013)

Welsh, Jennifer. "Researchers Who Provided Key Evidence For Gluten Sensitivity Have Now Thoroughly Shown That It Doesn't Exist." *Business Insider.* 15 May 2014. Web. http://www.businessinsider.com/gluten-sensitivity-and-study-replication-2014-5#ixzz3diU0WK9o

Chapter 19.
The Lowly Potato

What if I could tell you about a new wonder supplement?

What if I could tell you that the amino acid profile of this wonderful new supplement is as good or better than the best whey protein, calorie for calorie?

What if I could show you that this new wonder supplement has a higher biological value than soy protein as well – but it is also from a plant source?

Oh, and to make this new wonder supplement even healthier... what if I make sure the micronutrients of this new supplement is rich in Vitamin C and zinc, as well as B vitamins (both of these important for anabolic processes of tissue building) and also potassium, antioxidants, and even fiber for digestive efficiency?

Sounds pretty amazing, right?

You see how the mind works.

If I talk about this profile of a supplement, everyone is all ears and interested. But if I tell you this actually the nutritional profile of… a potato, well you're less interested, because potato is, well, just a potato. And it's a starch, and that can't be good for you.

But honestly, the potato is one of nature's best whole food suppliers.

In fact, if I just gave you a list of the nutritional composition of a potato – nutritional density, satiety index rating (which we will discuss below), amino acid and micronutrient profile – then you would see that the potato is not just a starchy carb, but an incredible wonder food. If I just gave you the list of its composition, without telling you the name of the food, you would want it in your diet.

There is much more that can be said of the power of the potato. In fact, you could live indefinitely on a diet of just potatoes if you had to, which is pretty rare for a single food item. That is how complete this food source is.

In fact this has been done over and over again in the past.

Danish physician and nutritionist Mikkel Hindhede in the 19th century tested his hypothesis that potatoes might be used to stave off famine, back when famine was a real issue. He lived off of mostly potatoes (with a little milk and butter) for several months. Not only did he live off a potato diet… he thrived on it as well. His own conclusion was, "Man can retain full vigor for a year or longer on a diet of potatoes and fat."

In an attempt to confirm or refute Hindhede's findings, a decade later Polish researchers Stanislaw Kon and Aniela Klein also went on an all potatoes diet for 167 days (with some coffee and some fruit). Special notes were made that digestion was "excellent" throughout the experiment, and Kon even maintained his athletic training schedule during the diet as well.

Suffice it to say there was a time in nutritional history when the potato was held out to be more or less a "nutritional hero" of sorts, the kind of status reserved today for manufactured supplements and acai berry drivel. I doubt anyone would or could go half a year on an all acai berries diet.

And yet there is even *more* to the history of this tremendous tuber. The first great South American civilization thrived because of cultivation of the potato. History shows that other potato-enabled civilizations followed, including the Incas, for whom two core staple foods were central to their survival – potatoes, and maize... *both* starches.

Historically we see the nutritional superhero status of the potato across Europe as well, and population growth followed everywhere that potato farming grew, from Switzerland to China.

Of course, it is also well-documented that the lowly potato led to the survival and thriving of the Irish. Once the potato became the chief source of caloric energy in the Irish diet, their population doubled during that century, and it practically doubled yet again in the 50 years following that. By the early- to mid-9th century, one in three Irish lived on virtually an all potato diet. When a fungus wiped out the potato crops, the great potato famine of Ireland from 1845-1852 led to one million dead from the famine, and another million who emigrated to escape it.

Now imagine any of the people from these eras of history, where their families thrived and survived with the potato as their staple food—imagine trying to convince *them* that potatoes are bad and unhealthy, and that they should stay away from them!

Oh, and from a "go Green" perspective as well, agriculturally, today the potato yields more food energy per planted acre than any other thing plant – another "plus" speaking to its superior nutritional and life-support status.

Yet because of modern fad diet nonsense that started with Atkins, and continued with Paleo, the potato has gone from Superhero to Superzero. That is insane. If you look at things clearly, this makes no sense, and the bias against the potato simply doesn't stand up to academic scrutiny.

For example, although the potato gets a bad rap because of its "glycemic index," something you seldom hear much about is **The Satiety Index**. When it comes to The Satiety Index, once again the potato becomes a "Superhero" of modern nutrition.

The Satiety Index and the Potato

Susanna Holt of the University of Sydney Australia did a research experiment in 1995 to compare the effects of different foods on short-term satiety and appetite levels.

She prepared 240 calorie portions of 38 different foods. These foods ran the gamut from yogurt to Mars Bars, to eggs, fruits, cheese, brown rice, ice-cream, candy—and yes... potatoes. Holt recruited volunteers and asked them to eat a single, 240 calories portion of each of the 38 foods, all on separate occasions of course.

After consuming each food, participants were then asked to rate their hunger levels every 15 minutes for the next two hours. From *there*, the participants were led to a buffet where they could eat as much or as little as they desired. Holt then counted the number of calories the participants ate in these follow-up meals, and she then combined this with the data she recorded regarding their previously reported hunger ratings from the participants' consumption of the 240 calorie portions of foods they ate prior to the buffet.

She used all this to create a "satiety index" for each of the 38 foods she was looking at. Now, just like the glycemic index, she also used white bread as her reference food and assigned it a score of 100. From there she summarized a food's satiation value, something seldom ever discussed in modern nutrition fields.

And the highest and best satiety index score was achieved by – yes indeed — *THE POTATO!* (Oh, and by a vast margin, I might add!)

The satiety index score she assigned to the potato was 323.

No other food was even close.

The second closest food was "ling fish" which scored 225. In other words, no other food came close to the potato in terms of leaving participants feeling "satisfied" after eating, or in terms of REDUCING the amount of food they ate a few hours later at the buffet.

Don't you think this is important when considering modern nutrition, metabolism and weight-control?

Foods with stronger short-term satiation effects are going to have more beneficial effects on appetite control over the course of the day. You would of course expect that people who eat more foods that don't provide much satiation to be heavier and have a harder time controlling appetite than people who eat foods with a higher satiation effect.

Other studies are indeed confirming this hypothesis: people who choose whole foods with a higher satiety value correlates with using such foods "as staples" for long-term weight control.

Why isn't anyone talking about this?

I would guess it is because the potato is a starch – a food category demonized as a matter of our modern cultural creation. Furthermore, the potato is a high glycemic food... so it can't be good for us, right? Talk about throwing the baby out with the bath water!

Let's talk about the relevance of the "glycemic index" here for a minute, shall we? The fitness and diet industry love their buzz words. The term "glycemic index" became entrenched in the low-carb argument, and many a healthy whole food was demonized as part of that argument—none more than the potato it seems.

"Everyone knows you shouldn't eat any starch that is white, after all!"

Please.

Cultures all over the world and throughout history knew from their own sense of biofeedback that potatoes were good for them.

The glycemic index is a faulty 'idea' attempting to replace reality. Moreover, it is an 'idea' thrown around by people who barely understand it. Oh sure, it sounds scientific. Good enough, right? According to this line of juvenile thinking, any and all high-glycemic foods are bad. The lowly potato was caught in the web of this "all-or-nothing," non-sensical logic.

The question I've always had is this: are there really any "unhealthy" unprocessed whole foods, that come from a plant source? I mean, really folks.

It's amazing how many research studies lump potatoes in with comments regarding French fries. This is akin to saying grass-fed skinless chicken breast is unhealthy, while making reference to KFC. Evidence continues to mount of the "re-discovered" superiority of the potato – despite the hangover of Atkins, Paleo and the rest of this nonsense.

A Protest Against the Potato That Didn't Work So Well

Back in 2011, as a protest against school lunches wanting to limit "starchy vegetables" by comparing all of them to French fries, the head of the Washington Potato Commission, Chris Voigt, like his 19th-century counterparts, went on all potato diet to illustrate the healthiness of potato.

Voigt's point was that it is fried oils, and frying the potatoes, that does all the harm.

Before his experiment, no one was listening, and his voice was going unheard in the backlash of pop-culture and ignorance informed by the likes of Atkins and Paleo. So Voigt took matters into his own hands and undertook a potatoes-only diet. **He ate nothing but potatoes, a whopping 20 of them per day, without topping, and he went for 60 straight days (over 8 weeks, folks).**

Now according to Paleo Preaching Pundits and Atkins Aficionados, two months of a pure starch diet should certainly cause Mr. Voigt to gain lots of fat, especially if his choice was the lowly potato, and especially if he was eating 20 of them per day! (Oh and let's not forget that he should also be "very afraid" that he may be become "insulin-resistant" by this eight week long all-potato potato diet.)

But what ACTUALLY happened?

Well, with over 60 days on the all starch, all potato

protest diet, Mr. Voigt *LOST* 21 lbs.

As for health indices? His cholesterol and triglyceride levels dropped significantly as well, and even his resting blood glucose levels improved (note this last one, as all these ill-advised anti-carb approaches to weight loss and weight-control love to malign the potato for its effects on blood glucose).

And just like the two researchers from the 19th century mentioned in Part 1, Mr. Voigt did not experience any loss of energy or productivity from his all potato diet.

Symptoms like weakness, loss of energy, lack of productivity, and scatter-brained attention spans, and so on — these are the most common reported side-effects of low-carb approaches.

Now, to be clear, I'm not saying to go out and go on an all potato diet. Any diet of severe food limitation make no sense, since it's not normal for our omnivore brains to be limited to one food. (We are not Koala Bears.) But still, a point about the superiority of the potato had to be made and Mr. Voigt made it!

Myself, I eat baked potatoes as my dinner starch source two to three times per week.

Demonizing the potato because of one single criterion like the glycemic index simply makes no sense and borders on the ridiculous. It totally lacks any consideration of context. When you consider the potato's stellar nutrient profile, its crucial role in the development of sustaining various cultures throughout history, and its satiation effects, and its effect on appetite-control and weight-control... well, the only conclusion you can possibly come to is that the potato is a modern whole unprocessed SUPERHERO SUPERFOOD if that label ever deserved to apply to any food source!

Chapter References

Drewnowski, Adam, and Colin D Rehm. "Vegetable Cost Metrics Show That Potatoes and Beans Provide Most Nutrients Per Penny." PLoS ONE 8.5 (2013): e63277. Web.

Gordon, Edgar S, Marshall Goldberg, and Grace J Chosy. "A New Concept in the Treament of Obesity." JAMA: The journal of the American Medical Association 186.1 (1964): 156–163. Print.

Holt, S H et al. "A Satiety Index of Common Foods." European journal of clinical nutrition 49.9 (1995): 675–690. Print.

Hindhede, M. "Vegetarian Experiment with a Population of 3 Million." JAMA :The journal of the American Medical Association 74.6 (1996): n. pag. Print.

Kon, Stanisław Kazimierz, and Aniela Klein. "The Value of Whole Potato in Human Nutrition." Biochemical Journal 22.1 (1928): 258–260. Print.

Reader, John. Potato: A History of the Propitious Esculent. New Haven: Yale UP, 2011. Print.

Chapter 20.
The Truth About Coffee

As I sit here drinking my venti Columbian blend, I recall how I wanted to write this article some two years ago when two contradictory research findings about coffee came through the news cycle within a week of each other.

One study "concluded" that coffee drinking could lead to ill-health, while the other one stated that coffee consumption undoubtedly promotes better health.

There is so much conflicting information it so often seems like… what's the truth?

Here's the thing:

The overall research for the last 20 years or so has been VERY CLEAR on coffee!

The research overwhelmingly **supports** coffee drinking as a potential health-promoting beverage. There actually really isn't much debate about where the overwhelming mountain of evidence is regarding coffee and health.

But oh how the media loves its research scare tactics and making people "afraid" of pretty much anything "enjoyable" these days. So let me spell it all out for you in this article (just after I grab my *second* morning cup of venti Columbian blend, thank you).

The Health and Physical Effects of Coffee

It's no secret of course that coffee heightens alertness and also increases athletic performance. That fact has never been in dispute. Caffeine improves speed and strength by accelerating the transmission of electrical signals from the brain to the muscles.

It improves endurance by reducing perceived effort, allowing for things like marathon running to feel easier. And of course it can also have positive situational metabolic effects and increase fat burning via mobilization and use of free fatty acids.

Indeed, there is now pretty much a library's worth of overwhelming evidence illustrating coffee's health promoting and other positive effects.

I just want to go through the "short-list" of beneficial physiological effects of coffee/caffeine consumption that are well-known, before I move on to the lesser-known research about the health benefits of your morning legal stimulant.

- Research is quite clear that caffeine from coffee increases the amount of fat burned during exercise. In active people, coffee can boost metabolism by as much as 15%. As indicated above, coffee/caffeine can increase adrenalin, so it is a great training aid – especially for a trainee in a depleted or exhausted state.

- Furthermore, for hard-training trainees, caffeine prevents exercise-induced decreases in intramuscular potassium; this means it keeps cells hydrated, and cell hydration promotes anabolic activity.

- As mentioned above, caffeine also increases the bioavailability of free fatty acids. This is important because this can spare glycogen. And sparing glycogen not only lends to prolonged higher performance, it also spares muscle protein because spared glycogen results in a delay of gluconeogenesis (using protein for energy.) And this also keeps cells hydrated.

- Research shows that in the presence of caffeine muscles use half as much glycogen during exercise because of increased use of intramuscular triglycerides. In one study, athletes were able to exercise for 96 minutes before they reached exhaustion, as compared to athletes taking a placebo who were exhausted after just a little over

70 minutes.

- That is a dramatic increase in performance and work capacity. In this study, gluconeogenesis was reduced by 55% among those taking caffeine. This spares both protein and carbohydrates, as well.

It is quite clear from the research that any trainee seeking an edge in performance and adaptation because of increased performance are "enhanced" by caffeine intake, particularly caffeine assimilated via coffee consumption.

(But as usual: let's not be idiots here – "more" isn't necessarily better, either.)

Other Correlations with Coffee Consumption

So it is pretty obvious that trainees interested in enhancing physique and performance would do well to become coffee consuming connoisseurs. But there are other correlations in research that suggest the health and wellness promotive effects of coffee consumption.

Lets' take a look at some this 'peer-reviewed' research below, because in many corners of the health and nutrition industry, coffee and caffeine continue to be considered "unhealthy" even though the truth in the vast majority of studies paints a different picture.

- One such study showed that coffee drinkers were less likely to commit suicide than the average person. In 1996, a Harvard study showed that heavy coffee drinkers were up to 40% less likely to kill themselves.

- In 2011, researchers from Harvard's School of Public Health reported that habitual coffee drinkers were up to 20% less likely to suffer from depression than were people who did not drink coffee.

In fact, over the last 20 years or so, research has certainly seemed to settle the matter about coffee consumption and its relation to health, and it settled IN FAVOR of coffee as a health-promoting indulgence. Research has shown that coffee drinkers are healthier than non-drinkers in many distinct ways.

Moreover, it seems that the heaviest consumers of coffee seem to benefit the most.

Research is pretty clear that coffee beasts like myself are less likely than others to develop heart disease, diabetes, dementia, specific types of cancers, liver disease, Parkinson's Disease, and as mentioned, depression.

One study suggests coffee drinkers may even out-live non coffee drinkers. A 2012 study published in The New England Journal of Medicine found that, within a population of more than 400,000 men and women, regular coffee consumers were 10% less likely to die during a 13-year observation period. What's also important to point out here is that it's not just the caffeine content of coffee that enhances health, but also its anti-oxidants, something that seldom gets much attention in discussions of coffee intake.

So… why do we still hear about the "controversy" of coffee?

This contradictory research that suggests coffee and caffeine are "bad" – where does it come from, and is it accurate?

In spite of the overwhelming evidence of the benefits of coffee drinking and the superior health and well-being observations of people who drink coffee, there are still experts who reject any notion of positive effects from coffee consumption, and these "experts" are usually part of some kind of diet zealotry.

For example, misinformed proponents of The Candida Diet, Detox Diets, various cleanses, and even The Zone Diet and the Atkins Diet forbid, warn against, or advise very strict limits on coffee consumption. *"Tea good – coffee bad!"* But beneath it all is this age old North American Diet Mentality suspicion that things people consume for pleasure "can't be good for you."

Now, let me explain where and how "anti-coffee crusaders" get off track.

One recent study on the ill-effects of coffee simply didn't hold up upon deeper investigation. The study suggested that people who drink 8 or more cups of coffee per day (me, for example!) were less healthy in a variety of ways than those who didn't drink much or any coffee at all. (Published in Mayo Clinic Review 2013) However, upon closer review of this research a different explanation surfaced.

It seems this had more to do with very speculative correlation than causation. It turned out that the people of the sample group observed in this study — those who drank that much coffee — well these subjects also seemed to be people who smoked, who drank alcohol regularly, who didn't exercise much, who didn't eat well, and who reported working long hours, eating fast food, and/or having stressful jobs and lives.

So upon closer inspection coffee consumption as a stimulant was merely an indicator of a deeper issue, and not a "causative" factor at all.

For coffee connoisseurs like myself, who do not have stressful lives, who eat well, exercise, take care of our bodies and don't use recreational drugs or alcohol and don't smoke – well this "unhealthy profile of coffee drinkers" simply disappears.

This is how "reductionist" research is often twisted to produce a specific message over an actual finding. What is missed in all of this "science" is the human experience with any food. I myself will continue to drink my morning coffee because of how I relate to the experience of doing so.

I have never bought into this silly modern notion that any enjoyable food or taste experience must be bad for me. I enjoy my daily coffee immensely.

And for all the reasons explained above, I suggest you do as well… "for the pure health of it!"

Chapter References

Abnet, CC. et al, "Association of coffee drinking with total and cause-specific mortality." New England Journal of Medicine, May 2012

Cano-Marquina, A. et al, "The impact of coffee on health" *Maturitas*, May, 2013

Duhon, J. et al, "Effect of caffeine RPE and perceptions of pain, arousal, and pleasure/displeasure during a cycling time trial in endurance trained and active men" *Physiology and Behavior*, May, 2012

Duncan, M.J and Oxford, SW. "Acute caffeine ingestion enhances performances and dampens muscle pain following resistance exercise to failure" *Journal of Sports Medicine and Physical Fitness*, June, 2012

Lucas, M. et al, "Coffee, caffeine, and risk of depression among women." *Archives of Internal Medicine*, Sept, 2011

Willett WC et al, "A prospective study on coffee drinking and suicide in women." *Archives of Internal Medicine*, March 1996

Chapter 21.
Artificial Sweeteners

Some time ago on my Facebook page I made a post regarding the 'non-issue' of the use of artificial sweeteners. The attack dogs came out in full force. One of the comments was that I was clearly "not up" on the research.

The problem here is that it's real research that matters. That's what I try to be "up on." There are certain things that define real research. For example, it must be peer-reviewed, and it must be replicable. Anything less than that is "junk science."

With the objectivity taken out of research in this industry it's hard to argue with people who have an agenda. Most people look at Big Pharma and think its responsible for manipulating people. The real irony is that since the Dietary Supplement Health Education Act of 1994 (DSHEA), it is actually the health food and supplements industries who are in a conspiracy to manipulate consumers and buy off politicians. For more on this, see Dan Hurley's book *Natural Causes: Death, Lies and Politics in America's Vitamin and Herbal Supplement Industry*.

Let's get to the issue of artificial sweeteners shall we?

For the record, I use them.

You could even say I use a lot of them.

I also consider myself a very healthy person who takes good care of my body. But instead of just quoting a bunch of research only to have people bark back at me with other research, usually junk science, I decided to simply seek out the real experts and get their opinions firsthand. This is what they had to say, mixed in with my own commentary as well.

The Usual Fear-Mongering Hype

In regards to artificial sweeteners, we hear everything from cancer to Alzheimer's to blood sugar issues, brain impairment and everything in-between as far as 'dangers' correlated with their use. But in truth, there isn't any link between artificial sweeteners and any of these in the real research.

One study gave rats *four hundred times* the amount of sweetener that any human would likely ever ingest (when adjusted for size and bodyweight), and the animals had no real side effects. Shocking.

Dr. Joe Schwarcz, director of the McGill University Center for Science and Society has been studying sweeteners and their supposed risks for years. He is also fully aware of the junk science involved in creating false fears. He's quite emphatic that the human data simply do not show a link between ill-health and sweeteners. Here's what he had to say:

> "Of course you can find the odd study that raises an eyebrow. But this is often because of what is known as a 'positive finding bias.' In other words, a study that shows or even hints at a link between sweeteners and ill-health – these studies get all the press. But what the public doesn't realize is that these findings aren't duplicated in other studies – and being able to duplicate findings is one of the cornerstones of real and true scientific research."

You see, in this fast-paced digital world of news and the media competing for consumer attention, fear-raising and "warning" stories make good news. These kinds of studies make the rounds on news feeds and websites often before they are even verified or confirmed, and often without the full study being given for context.

Even reputable health-care organizations sometimes get it wrong in their rush to want to be first. In the fall of 2012 esteemed Brigham's Women's Hospital Boston stood behind a study suggesting that artificial sweeteners like aspartame raise the risk of leukemia and lymphoma. This initial endorsement by such a prestigious establishment lent significant weight to the anti-sweetener brigade. But only one week later, the hospital recanted the endorsement, stating that it had been "premature in promoting this evidence." But of course, by then, it was too late as the internet and marketing forces had already latched on to the endorsement.

Around the same time a U.S. population study linked the consumption of diet soft drinks to an increased risk of heart attack, stroke, and cardiac death, and the immediate leap was made that sweeteners were the culprit. But University of Ottawa obesity specialist Dr. Yoni Freedhoff said of the study, "This study is worthless and shows a glaring failure of peer review." Dr. Freedhoff also offered this: "If the choice is between sugar and sweetener in patients trying to manage their weight for health-reasons, there is no doubt, and no question, that the current state of the evidence would be in favor of using the sweeteners, of course."

As far as this new claim that aspartame interferes with brain function, this claim has been at best wishy washy and "theoretical." Dr. Ronnie Aronson, the medical director of LMC Diabetes and Endocrinology in Toronto, said this about the risks of aspartame interfering with brain function: "A large body of literature for both children and adults has found no cause for concern about these sweeteners" (excluding people of course who have PKU, which is a genetic disorder to do with the intake of the amino acid phenylalanine). Dr. Aronson continued, "In one such study, military pilots exposed to high levels of aspartame were given a series of complex cognitive tests, which showed no ill effects whatsoever."

Stevia

There are also those who will look kindly on a sweetener if it comes from a natural source, because anything else that's man-made must be dangerous, right?

Dr. Joe Schwarcz finds this line of reasoning as illogical as I do. His comment was, "Whether something is safe to consume or not, or is healthy or not, has nothing to do with whether it comes from a lab or a bush. You must beware of the common fallacy of equating natural to good, and artificial to bad."

A note on that fallacy: I am slightly guilty of this, as I argued earlier in this very book that there are certain unnatural aspects of our modern world that are having a very negative effect on our metabolisms. But I actually still stand by that argument. It's not so much that I'm simplistically saying "natural: good… unnatural: bad!" My point, rather, is that our body is not equipped to "naturally" deal with our modern environment of abundance, and the environmental cues for the rewarding foods which surround us. We are also not "naturally" equipped to deal with the hyper-palatable foods made up of sugar, salt, and fat, that have been engineered in labs precisely to light up the reward centers of our brains.

I absolutely still stand by that argument. And when you consider that argument, then you compare an artificial sweetener to something "natural" like Stevia or to *actual sugar*, it's obvious which one is going to have the greater effect on the brain's reward centers and induce greater cravings. You can also tell which one will have the less desirable effect on insulin, metabolism, and so on.

Moreover, the argument that "natural sources are better" with respect to Stevia *also* falls apart when you consider the following: sugar cane is a natural plant, but it has to go to the factory to be processed into table sugar. Likewise, Stevia still has to be harvested and also sent to the factory where it too must be "processed" in order to be available on store shelves. It is not much different as a processed food condiment than is any other prepared artificial sweetener out there. Maple syrup is very natural coming from the sap of the maple tree, if you can get it from a small business in Ontario or Quebec or something. But normally, it too must go to the factory to be processed into maple syrup if you're going to find it on grocery store shelves. At the end of the day, these are still "sugars" that most people try to avoid, for good reason.

To think Stevia is somehow "superior" just feeds some prideful "healthier than thou" type of thinking.

But that said...

There is a danger with artificial sweeteners that has to do with calorie counting.

Don't kid yourself that because you are using "sweetener" over here, it frees up calories for other food *over there*.

This is known as compensatory behavior or psychological negotiation. Yes, using sweeteners can save you calories, but it saves you the "extra" calories that you didn't need anyway. It doesn't mean you need to go get more calories from other sources. This is wishful thinking. Remember: manage realistic expectations.

I don't use sweeteners as a calorie savings strategy, in that I don't think that way. I use sweeteners just because I don't want the metabolic effects of what "sugar" would do in my body if I ate it. But since I've *always* had a sweet tooth, and that's been ingrained in me by my upbringing (we had a lot of sweet snacks when I was a kid) there is no dilemma for me in solving this with the use of an artificial sweetener alternative.

Remember that a diet must be sustainable longterm. In a world where we *have* been exposed to hyper palatable foods, and we do have those sugar cravings, artificial sweeteners are a reasonable component of a sustainable diet strategy. That is why artificial sweeteners have earned a place in my diet.

To summarize, artificial sweeteners do not have the same deleterious nutrient-partitioning effects and metabolic consequences that actual sugar and its variations does.

I agree with Dr. Freedhoff's claim that given the state of the evidence of "real" science, if it's a choice between sugar and artificial sweeteners for my everyday nutritional fare… I choose sweeteners!

Chapter References

Grice, H C, and L A Goldsmith. "Sucralose--an Overview of the Toxicity Data." *Food and Chemical Toxicology* 38 (Suppl. 2) (2000): S1–S6. Print.

I also recommend Dr. Yoni Freedhoff's blog: http://www.weightymatters.ca/ — he regularly posts peer-reviewed research studies with commentary on their validity and the context in which they should be considered (such as who's paying for the study, what variables are left out, and so on) and has several posts discussing studies on artificial sweeteners.

Chapter 22.
How to Spot Diet Scams

It seems odd to end a book with a chapter like this, but I think it appropriate. If you've read this far, you probably know my position on the simplicity of what it takes to maintain and promote a healthy metabolism. There is elegance in simplicity, and simple doesn't mean easy. The more complicated a system or diet is, the less likely it is to actually be good for metabolic function.

Between ads for Nutrisystem, Herbal Magic and the plethora of infomercials and all the rest, we're now at a point where everyday major brands and marketers will lie directly to your face about the science of weight-loss and metabolism, over-complicating it and over-promising what they can deliver.

Companies and fitness gurus lie about the science of weight-loss because they can't talk to you about the likelihood of you achieving it. They also co-opt what are actually reasonable, healthy messages and use them for their own ends. Like any good hucksters, they use a little bit of truth, a dash of hyperbole, and a bunch of misinformation to sell you something you are already psychologically primed to buy into, because they're selling to our innermost desires.

Let's look at a few of the warning signs to look for when trying to sniff out the nonsense of weight-loss scams.

1.

Suggestions that weight-loss will be quick, easy and linear.

No changes of any kind that adults make are quick and easy. *None*!

Think about it: a change in relationship status, a change in job, a move to a new city—none of these are "quick and easy."

This speaks to the psychology of change in adults. All kinds of studies show that adult brains are more resistant to change than are children's. This is why it's easier to learn another language as a child than as an adult. And a change that involves physiological change is going to be even more non-linear, with a lot of back and forth involved because the adult body, like the adult mind, resists change as well.

Change like this is possible, but it is not easy or linear. Accept it, and be wary of anything or anyone that promises otherwise.

2.

Diets that emphasize one food or food group or one macronutrient.

Everything from low fat, to low carbs and all their variations including Paleo and the rest.

This kind of emphasis makes "honeymooning" on these diets very easy, because of the anti-catabolic phase of weight loss, and the psychology of them, but the reality of sustaining them? Not so much. Almost always these diets create some kind of imbalance over time. Furthermore, these tend to be the kinds of diets that demonize certain macronutrient groups, even healthy whole foods (e.g. "Wheat Belly"). If you see that, run far.

3.

Claims that you can eat all you want and still lose weight.

This is the kind of infomercial nonsense still floating around, catering to desire and fantasy, but not reality. People don't want the truth, they want some fantastical version of it.

I even have a diet that promises a daily cheat day (or even a cheat day plus a mid week spike in some cases) but that only works in a very specific metabolic environment called "supercompensation," and I'm very up front about this.

Diets that do imply you can eat what you want are catering to the exact part of your brain that keeps you struggling with weight in the first place. It's impossible to "eat all you want and still lose weight." IMPOSSIBLE.

In fact, the opposite is often true. You have to retrain your mind to actually *"want* to eat less." (Your goal is tolerable hunger.) That is diet-psychology reality.

4.

Guaranteed lasting results.

Again, this is just nonsense catering to our own wish bias. How can any company or service guarantee lasting results for something that boils down to a matter of your own personal responsibility, behavioral consistency, and commitment?

Anything that implies that your own behavior, commitment, and responsibility are not necessary or an important part of "lasting results" is just lying. There are no guarantees that anyone but you can offer, because programs only work when YOU work them. No outside force can guarantee that YOU will stick to doing what needs to be done to secure "changes that last forever."

5.

Claims that dealing with food sensitivities and

allergies will "cure" your weight issues.

Gluten "sensitivity," carb "resistance" and such come to mind. This one particularly bothers me.

I mentioned in other chapters that some people have slower metabolisms, or are starting a few years back from the regular start line. But this food sensitivity and allergy stuff doesn't count. It bothers me because it caters to a "victim" mindset, and that is just about the least empowering mindset any human being can adopt. Being overweight is not "caused" by sensitivities and allergies to food. That makes no sense in biochemical reality. What it does is pander to the victim mindset, and we have far too much of that in this society already.

If you have food allergies or sensitivities, fine. Those are real! Deal with them. But don't pretend that this is what led you to be overweight, or to stay that way!

6.

Claims that 'our' diet combined with 'our' supplements burn off the fat.

Really, Jillian? Really, Herbal Magic? Really Isagenics? Body by V? Lipozene?

The shelves are filled with fat burners, and if any one of them worked, *they would put all the other ones out of business in within a month.*

There are no known supplements that speed fat burning or burn fat in the permanent sense. Caffeine is the only thing that comes close, but even with caffeine, making such a direct claim would be misleading.

Any supplements that go along with a calorie restriction diet are just plain riding on the coat tails of the calorie restriction. It's the calorie restriction doing the work. Fat burner supplements are useless. Period.

7.

Cleanses, fasts, HCG Injections, BodyWraps, Vibration Machines, herbs and cellulite treatments.

Ads for these gimmicks as part of sustainable weight-control are scraping the bottom of the barrel and usually appeal to the most desperate. None of these things will have any bearing on long-term sustainable weight-loss, and you should run as fast as you can away from anyone promoting such nonsense.

8.

Secret Breakthrough Findings.

Psychologists have shown that certain buzzwords like this appeal to the attention centers of our brains and get us to pay attention to whatever is being said after that word has been used.

Here's the truth: there haven't really been "breakthroughs" in weight-loss research in decades, so we need to stop pretending there is a weight-loss Santa Claus. He ain't real, folks.

If there are any secrets, it's the research going on in

academia that shows what we've known all along: if you want to lose weight, you'll have to be consistent, you'll be a bit hungry, and you won't get to eat whatever you want—and at the same time, going for "extremes" will always backfire in the end.

These are only a few ways to spot diet scams that come to my mind right now. They are the most obvious and common ones. You need to tell yourself that anyone using these tactics is not looking out for your best interests, they are looking out for their own.

Learn More

To learn more about diet, training, and physique transformation, or to get announcements about future books, please visit my website and subscribe to my email list: **http://scottabelfitness.com/**. I send out free articles on nutrition and working out, as well as case studies, client updates, and more.

If you liked this book, and want to see more, please take a moment to **write a review on Amazon** and let me know! (I'd actually really appreciate it.)

Thank you for purchasing and taking the time to read this book!

ALL RIGHTS RESERVED. No part of this publication may be reproduced or transmitted in any form whatsoever, electronic, or mechanical, including photocopying, recording, or by any informational storage or retrieval system without express written, dated and signed permission from the author.

DISCLAIMER AND/OR LEGAL NOTICES: Every effort has been made to accurately represent this book and it's potential. Results vary with every individual, and your results may or may not be different from those depicted. No promises, guarantees or warranties, whether stated or implied, have been made that you will produce any specific result from this book. Your efforts are individual and unique, and may vary from those shown. Your success depends on your efforts, background and motivation.

The material in this publication is provided for educational and informational purposes only and is not intended as medical advice. The information contained in this book should not be used to diagnose or treat any illness, metabolic disorder, disease or health problem. Always consult your physician or health care provider before beginning any nutrition or exercise program. Use of the programs, advice, and information contained in this book is at the sole choice and risk of the reader.

Made in the USA
Lexington, KY
08 October 2015